EVERYTHING THEY DON'T TEACH AT HARVARD MEDICAL SCHOOL

H

A DIET FOR A LITTLE PLANET

BENJAMIN SARLIN M.D. M.S.

10 STEPS TO HEALTH GREATNESS

Acknowledgements

B'H"

Thank you to all those who supported me on this book, G-d, my family, friends, Rabbis, editors Brittany Horwitt, Sandy Leschen, others who helped, and most to those in LA.

"Put yourself on a single meal a day, now--dinner--for a few days, till you secure a good, sound, regular, trustworthy appetite, then take to your one and a half permanently, and don't listen to the family any more. When you have any ordinary ailment, particularly of a feverish sort, eat nothing at all during twenty-four hours. That will cure it. It will cure the stubbornest cold in the head, too. No cold in the head can survive twenty-four hours' unmodified starvation."
-Mark Twain

What are they focusing on? The symptoms, how to prevent the outcome...We're not focusing on the underlying philosophy or approach. A person who is ill can be healed in one of two ways. One way is to wait until he is in grave danger, and then begins to seek a remedy, or he can be sent to the hospital where he will be confined, due to his unstable condition, for he is unhinged. Then there is the correct approach. This is from the start to ensure that "all the illnesses I sent that I visited upon Egypt will not befall you". This must cause us to change our approach to education of belief in one's own strength. When the education of youth is based on a creator who gives you strength, who gives you life, then when he is taught on this foundation, we will do away with the need to heal and won't arrive at this situation of unhealthy children and students.
-Rebbe Menachem Mendl Schneerson

"Unless someone like you cares a whole awful lot, nothing is going to get better. It's not."
-Dr. Seuss

CONTENTS

1 Everything They Don't Teach at Harvard Medical School

My first year of medical school in Israel, I often studied in the Hilton Hotel overlooking the Mediterranean. As the rough waves of the sea swept over the shore outside, I was warm and quiet inside. I'd usually come for lunch and eat my favorite dish from the lobby restaurant, fish and chips. The country is a paradigm of irony, modern and Ancient, sweet and bitter, spiritual and material. Full of world-class hotels, half the country lives in hunger. The character of the people there, foreign writers compare to a bitter fruit known as a "sabra", prickly on the outside, sweet on the inside. The hotel lobby sparkled with travelers from all over the world. Business people in designer suits made deals and singles dressed in black and white spoke quietly over sodas. The Asian staff in the sushi bar spoke in three languages mixing Hebrew, English, and Thai. Whereas, a hundred years ago, we may have been able to find a clear answer on diet and nutrition, today finding out what to eat for good health remains elusive. With global economies, intertwined cultures, and mixed meals, we get mixed messages.

There are many countries we could fly to for enlightenment. In Okinawa, one would observe sashimi, seaweed and sake, in Patagonia, mongo nuts, river trout and venison, and in the North Pole, caviar, and arctic snow goose. Asia is no longer "The Orient" surrounded in mystery. Israel remains the land of milk and honey, but fruits and vegetables appear from all over the world. As the foods in various nations have become more and more similar, every nation is really standing on a river, looking at a reflection of itself in the water. Where can we find a sensible answer for eating healthfully every day? Simple answers to complex problems come from simple places. Our best lessons on obesity and weight loss aren't found drinking wine on the Riviera, eating fruit on South Beach, or dipping sushi in Sydney. They aren't found in a secret vault below the Vatican, underneath the Alamo, or in a lost ark in the desert. They are right before our eyes. We like to believe the fat cell is a place we will never find, when in fact we are standing right on the river.

Mark Twain once wrote the following about the Mississippi River:

Apparently, nobody happened to want such a river, nobody needed it, nobody was curious about it; so, for a century and a half, the Mississippi remained out of the market and undisturbed. When De Soto found it, he was not hunting for a river, and had no present occasion for one; consequently he did not value it, or even take any particular notice of it.[i]

A similar thing might be said about Diabetes (high blood sugar) today. Popular periodicals spin the same news stories on cholesterol month after month much as Huck Finn, spins his new campaign to repaint the same white fence outside Tom's home. Meanwhile Diabetes is making its way in stealth through every town and neighborhood. Like Desoto and the Mississippi, it remains out of the market and undisturbed. High blood sugar is the primary cause of heart disease, obesity, blindness, kidney failure, and sexual dysfunction. We do not value this, or even take any particular notice of it.

Mark Twain once wrote that to be the first to discover something is the greatest source of happiness in life. But if one goes deeper, this discovery is only a source of happiness if one has the ability to share it with others. It is like the baseball player who spent his whole life trying to pitch a no-hitter. When he accomplished his lifelong dream, he sat alone after his victory, having never married in his pursuit of "victory." Could any such epiphany be more of a heartbreak as he sat with his head in hands crying on the bench in his loneliness? The real key to success and happiness when one achieves health and well-being is being able to share this with others. This is the basis for all successful weight loss programs, but many don't know the secret to this success. When it comes to making fat in the body, the recipe has been around since the 1960s. But for some reason, while the scientist defined the pathway, he did not see, value, or take notice of it. He made no effort to make his discovery widely known. He shared it with academia alone. And so it has remained undiscovered and out of the market, like the Mississippi. The answer is blowing in the wind.

At Harvard medical school, a few years ago, a student asked about the side effects of cholesterol medications. The Professor ridiculed and humiliated him. Immediately, the students sensed something was wrong. When they investigated, they found their Professor was a paid consultant to numerous drug companies, including nearly half a dozen makers of cholesterol drugs. He was paid tens of thousands a year by pharmaceutical companies for "consulting" on cholesterol. When the story broke, Harvard received an F grade in an ethics ranking of medical schools, from the American Medical Student Association, a ranking of how medical schools are influenced by drug industry finances.

Faculty members receive tens or even hundreds of thousands of dollars a year through so called "consulting" fees. Nearly 20% of Harvard professors and instructors now have a direct financial interest in a business related to their teaching, research, clinical medicine, or a family member with such an interest. Over 200 medical professors and scientists are supported by either Pfizer or Merck Pharmaceuticals.[ii][iii]

The larger lie though is that "Familial hypercholesterolemia" is even the cause of a heart attack. It is in fact a rare 1 in 2 million disorder. The disease is more rare than cystic fibrosis, hemochromatosis (iron overload), and diabetes combined. But as Mark Twain once wrote, "A truth is not hard to kill. A lie told well is immortal." Everything to be learned about obesity and heart disease they don't teach at Harvard Medical School.

This is much like the story of a British general leading the painstaking building of a bridge for the Japanese in World War II. He invests the very core of his being in designing and raising this bridge. And yet when the Allies come to liberate them, he's unwilling to blow up the enemy bridge. Many lives and careers have been built on cholesterol research. Changing an idea is easy in life. But admitting one was wrong is something at which the medical profession has never excelled. They refuse to blow up the bridge. And so the real river lies in hiding. Just as losing weight is no guaranty a person will be kind and compassionate, a ticket to Harvard Medical School is no guarantee that its medical student leaves with basic ethics and decency. When Professors are hired to be part of a pharmaceutical empire, they often wind up building bridges for the enemy and then refusing to blow them up when victory is declared.

When doctors speak of obesity and heart disease today, they love to use large words derived from Latin such as "caloric" or "Genetic." "Breast Cancer? Obesity? It's genetic", they'll say. When a doctor does not really know what causes a health problem, he or she usually refers to it as a genetic disease. Over 90% of major hospitals and medical colleges teach and practice caloric theory, a theory as vague and inexplicable to a high school student as the location of the Mississippi River. Writings on obesity today have one thing in common. They use varying narrative diversions to bring us continually further downstream from our destination. A few years before his passing Steve Jobs told students at Stamford University "Don't be trapped by dogma--- which is the results of other people's thinking. Don't let the noise of others' opinions drown out your inner voice. And most important, have the courage to follow your heart and intuition." Intuitive thinking and creativity are no guarantee for basic ethics and morals.

Since we have completed the entire code to the human Genome map, we are no closer to self-understanding, or understanding our major diseases. Since the genome discovery late last decade, not a single major disease is closer to being cured. It comes as less of a surprise when we understand that we don't even understand the basics of obesity. In the 1950s we found a cure for Polio and cracked the code for DNA. Fifty years later, we have satellites, space shuttles and smartphones. But the code inside the fat cell remains to be broken. In addition to a change of perspective, we need an answer for the simple question. How exactly is fat made inside a fat cell? We need the simple user's guide, close up, in focus, and in simple terms a high school student can understand. We are no closer to knowing ourselves and our enemy than 100 years ago. Having a map, genetic or otherwise, is of no great use if we don't even know we're standing.

2   Breaking through the Fat Code-- The Answer

Fat-making is not Quantum Mechanics. Understanding how we battle obesity, does not require building the smartphone in white spacesuits. It is an attainable concept and a clearly defined pathway. The molecule fat is not a minute particle, like an electron, suspended in a state of eternal mystery. It is not made from a calorie, a vague term for how much heat a food releases. Most discussions of calories, or even insulin, the fat storage hormone, have little bearing on what happens in a fat cell. We have to assume that the battle plan for fat design exists in someone's war room. And we have to believe the finite design for fat-making in the human body is really a solvable mystery. However, the dusty blueprint remains undiscovered like a pearl at the bottom of a deep blue sea. A fat cell remains like the river we are standing on, that remains to be discovered. How we get fat still remains a mystery today. Nature may be mysterious. But this is due to her modesty rather than her arrogance. If the fat cell were to be compared to one of the planets, it would probably lie somewhere beyond the farthest reaches of the galaxy. As for distant planets, they are something we know that exist, and telescopes can find them. Each year, we discover new stars and planets. Yet when it comes to how fat is made in our body, we have fallen asleep, like Rip Van Winkle under the apple tree. "How exactly is fat made in a fat cell?" Can someone even answer this, close up, in focus, and in simple terms a high school student can understand? In addition to a change of perspective, we desperately need an answer for this one very simple question yet unanswered. How exactly is fat made inside a fat cell?

Today the elementary school chalkboard on caloric theory that might look a little like this:

Fat : 9 calories per gram
Protein : 4 calories per gram
Sugar : 4 calories per gram.
Excess calories ➔   *Fat*

15

The current high school chalkboard tells us little to nothing. Calories may tell us the equivalent of how much heat or energy is provided by fat (oils and butter), carbohydrates (grains and fruits), or protein (meat and eggs). But does it tell us how fat is made? If someone asks you what color a duck is and you tell them it is the third color in the rainbow, you have answered the question, but it doesn't mean they can picture it. Most people accept caloric theory like it's a cute little duck that sounds nice being yellow. But have you ever looked at it? A duck isn't yellow. It's white. Fat is like a rubber duck we can't actually get our hands on. It's slippery and flies away every time we seem to get a grip on it.

The calorie is so opaque, so unclear, and so "scientific", that it has most adults convinced that it is the ultimate answer, a scientific constant, like the speed of light. But children can usually sense falseness where adults cannot. So when the doctor explains to the teenager why too many calories is the answer, you can see the child's eyes roll over. How is this an answer? You've said nothing that makes sense at all. Saying a calorie makes us fat is about as unspecific and as ungrounded as can be. It's like saying $E=MC$ squared is the cause of obesity. How can you even argue with it? At the end of the office visit, the doctor asks, "Would you like a lolly pop? The teenager simply rolls her eyes and delivers the line of this generation, "What –ever….."

We remain as a country suspended in these 1970s calorie-led guidelines, the equivalent of an eight track tape diet. This mode of thinking still permeates every major hospital and medical clinic. With caloric theory we are still stuck with an inaccurate programming language and a flawed operating system. Only 17% of dieters say they follow a different approach from caloric theory, despite a decade of top works on insulin, the fat storage hormone, such as The Zone Diet. Medical schools like Harvard still do not consider insulin significant, because total fat calories determine how much fat is made in the fat cell, is the argument. Insulin just stores it. Their argument was not unfounded. It just is incorrect. Fat doesn't make us fat. The current health blueprint is really unchanged from thirty years ago. With caloric theory, we're still standing on the river.

The Answer: The Quick Users Guide

Grain, Fruit, Sugar →

Carbohydrate (starch) →

Glucose (sugar) →

Glycerol Phosphate (sugar derivative) →

Fat (Triglyceride)

Fat (Fatty Acids plus Glycerol) X ---(CANNOT) →
Fat (Triglyceride)

Exact pathway:

Grains or fruit →Carbohydrate (sugar or starch) →
Glucose (sugar) → acetyl Coa→ fatty acids
(With fatty acid synthase)

Grains or fruit →Carbohydrate (sugar or starch) →
Glucose (sugar) → glycerol 3 phosphate* (sugar
derivative) + fatty acids = adipose triglyceride or fat
(*Rate-limiting reagent)

Triglyceride (fat) → fatty acids + glycerol(recycled to
liver) ≠ adipose triglyceride or fat

But…..

Triglyceride (fat) → Glycerol → ≠ Triglyceride (Fat)

18

When fat enters the borders of a fat cell, it breaks into two parts glycerol and fatty acids. The two molecules then search around the fat cell to find one another. When they reunite, the glycerol extends his hand to the fatty acid. Try as they may, they never see one another again.[iv][v] Their hands only fall away. However, the fatty acid won't be disappointed. What's ready to greet it is glucose, in the form of glycerol phosphate. Sugar, transformed, carries off his fatty acid, and the two live happily ever after. Fat is simply masquerading. It plays no true part in fat production in the human body. Another way of viewing fat-making is that just as a plant builds fat in its seeds, from glucose and carbon dioxide, we humans do the same, with glucose.[vi] So what would happen if, theoretically, we consume a large quantity of dietary fat or oil? What if someone were to take a large container of olive oil and drink this? Or even better an entire vat of chicken fat? .[vii] [viii] Such a diet, consisting of entire bottles and vats of unlimited fat, therefore, has no ability to create body fat. The entire gallon of fat would lead to no weight gain or body fat, passing to the liver and being removed from the body. A source of triglyceride is continuous as long as there is a source of carbohydrate in the diet, whether from starch within whole grains, or simple sugars such as sucrose or glucose. Starch and sugar are the primary vehicles for fat production in the human body.[ix][x] The vast majority of carbohydrate is converted into body fat, not blood sugar. [xi]

One cannot download a song without proper punctuation in the website address, or send an email without periods in the right place. Similarly, one molecule turns out to be the difference between being able to make fat from sugar and not from fat. An email address without proper punctuation is an email that will never get to its destination. Fat is like a song that cannot be downloaded into our body, or like an email without the right punctuation to reach its intended destination. As far as our health goes, one phosphate molecule makes a world of difference. In Hebrew, the word mikreh, means chance, or a coincidence, happenstance. The same word mikrah, means "G-d is calling us [xii] Think one

19

letter doesn't make a difference? Science is not as Joseph Heller says, "A trash bag of random coincidence blown open in the wind", like calories and random sparks of fire thrown into a fat cell. Everything in the universe, from the peel of an apple, to the structure of a fat cell, is determined. Scientists simply got too complicated, turning obesity into quantum mechanics with random flying sparks of heat, to try to make it so the common person couldn't relate. It was an untested theory.

In simple terms, the carbohydrates in waffles and ice cream can make us fat. The fat in the waffles cannot. The carbohydrate in baked potatoes can make us fat, but not the butter or sour cream on top. The carbohydrate in a burger, fries, and soda can make us fat, but not the burger, the fat, or the frying oil. As anyone with Diabetes knows, it doesn't matter whether you eat a bowl of cheerios, a glass of juice or a few cookies, or candy bar. Your body doesn't care where the blood sugar comes from. All the talk of glycemic indexes and glycemic loads, with fancy mathematical calculations are just different shades of blue. If you have 10 grams of plutonium in a food, surrounded by lead, whether it is leaking slowly or quickly, doesn't matter. A Carbohydrate is like the toxic nuclear energy of the human body. Carbohydrate makes us fat, not fat itself. Grab a pen, and write it twenty times. Fat doesn't make you fat.

In the 1970s, the US government constructed a supposedly instructional food pyramid, a dietary plan that put grains and fruits on the pyramid's base, and meats and vegetables on top. Today, the pyramid is a "plate," but it makes little difference. The Food pyramid led to physicians and mainstream media encouraging a diet high in carbohydrates, contained in grains and fruit. According to one advertisement in New York by New York State's Department of Social services, a sign with a large burger reads, "Cut the Junk. Eating too much fried, fatty and fast food can bring on obesity, diabetes and heart disease. For more information on eating healthy and nutritious recipes, call 311 or visit nyc.gov. Perhaps the sign should say call 911. Because starch, not fat is the cause of obesity, diabetes and heart disease.

Recommended low-calorie diets, however, still today make no distinction between calories that come from fat and protein and those from sugar. Doctors encourage a low-fat (and low-calorie) diet, simply so as follow current hospital guidelines and rigid protocols. The recommendations make no distinction between calories from sugar, protein, and fat. They simply need to make Twinkies $8 a bag like cigarettes for kids to stop eating them. One in four children is obese. The other three are trying to avoid being trampled by them on the lunch line.

No animal eats grains whether a mammal or a sea mammal. They eat grass. Grains and fruits aren't found in the top 20 of total vitamins, minerals, or fiber. Breakfast cereal is made by carrying away the germ of the corn, destined for animal feed, and fiber, while the crystalline starch that remains is ground into pellets. Cheerios are nothing more than microcrystalline starch. Starch is a long molecule of glucose, which takes less than half a second to dissolve into simple sugars in the stomach. When this sugar enters the blood, it turns largely into fat. A tiny amount supplies the only organ that needs it, red blood cells. The rest damages arteries, and feeds cancer cells, which use only sugar for fuel. A low carbohydrate diet is the primary cure for Cancer today. Each gram of sugar in the diet courses into the blood at a rapid conversion to 3-5 points of blood sugar. The average American consumes 50 grams of sugar per meal, raising their blood sugar up to 250 points above baseline. (Normal is 60-90micrograms/dl) All this, when Protein (fish, meat, legumes) can break down into sugar and supply all the need for sugar needed by red blood cells. Fat cannot turn into sugar, and is used primarily to make the brain during childhood and to make hormones.

In the most famous experiment in Diabetes, the addition of table sugar to breakfast cereal surprisingly lowers the glucose and insulin responses to the meal! [xiii] [xiv] So ironically, if we were to dump out a whole bowl of breakfast cereal, such as cheerios, and replace it with table sugar, the insulin levels drop! A bowl of steel cut oats, the best grain on the planet, has 30 grams of carbohydrate as starch and four to five grams of fiber. There is no such thing as a complex carbohydrate. There is carbohydrate. And there is fiber. And the divide between them is as wide as an ocean. Yet steel-cut oats, with 30 grams of carbohydrate and 4 grams of fiber is somehow viewed as "complex". Yet a coca cola with 30 grams of carbohydrate is "simple". The carbohydrates are the same. But people again don't apparently see the Mississippi even if they are drinking it. Why is it that we see a food that is 10% fiber as complex? Who brainwashed us into thinking complex carbohydrates were 90% fiber when they are 90% starch. Whole oats or whole pearled rye are the best grains and yet they are still no better than 10% fiber. Five to six grams of fiber cannot magically make the starch in oats disappear.

When a child is fed a bowl of cheerios and glass of orange juice, he has just eaten the equivalent of a salad and a candy bar in terms of carbohydrates. But the salad combination has infinitely more nutrition, enzymes, vitamins, minerals, and fiber. The whole glycemic index (GI) and glycemic load is much like caloric theory, designed to make this concept more abstract, more scientific than it needs to be. Nevertheless, a candy bar has a lower GI than orange juice! (See p.25) And coca cola is lower than quaker oats. We need to stop feeding kids oatmeal and orange juice. It's like saying, let them eat cake. You wouldn't feed your kid a donut and coffee for breakfast. You wouldn't feed your kid a glass of wine and cigarettes for breakfast. Why do you feed yourself this way? Take a look at the glycemic index. A picture is worth a hundred words.

In the typical Western nation such as America today, 1 in 2 women and 1 in every 3 men are obese. More than 1 in every 2 black women is overweight.[xv] Carbohydrate consumption has increased dramatically to over 150 grams a day. The current American diet currently contains only 12% protein, less than a cow gets from grass and insects.[xvi] [xvii] [xviii] [xix] We're not insectivores, yet we get less protein than they do. If America was what we ate, we would be a bottle of Aunt Jemima. The National Health and Nutrition Examination Survey, conducted by the U.S. National Center for Health Statistics, reported its findings on food and consumption patterns in America. In 1983, the most consumed foods were white bread, rolls and crackers. In second, were donuts, cookies and cake. Alcoholic beverages came in third.[xx] Cereal grains contributed 31%, dairy products 14%, beverages 8%, oils and dressings 4%, and sugar and candy 4% of our diet. A decade later, the third National Health and Nutrition Examination Survey Number showed a similar pattern in popular foods for children. The most consumed foods were whole milk, chocolate milk, pizza, soft drinks, low-fat milk and cold cereal.[xxi] [xxii] Some predict that by mid century, 90% of children in the United States will be overweight. So much for everything in moderation.

Most body fat is made in a baby during the final three months of pregnancy. This occurs through the transfer of glucose to the infant and its primary use for body fat production.[xxiii] [xxiv] In 1954, scientists first wrote of the connection between "excessively large infants" and high blood sugar.[xxv] In 1977, Steven Gabbe wrote, "hyperglycemia [in the mother] may produce hyperinsulinemia and "macrosomia", or large birth weight babies." [xxvi] [xxvii] High carbohydrate intake is the major cause of overweight babies. The more obese the child, the more obese the adult. An overweight child is almost sure to be an overweight adult.[xxviii] After birth, infants are fed mother's milk. This milk is low in sugar (7 grams of every 100 grams of milk) and contains only one carbohydrate, lactose, which is broken down slowly. There is no starch, glucose, or fructose in mother's milk.[xxix] We don't feed babies orange juice, grape juice or oatmeal for a reason. Weight gain happens very rapidly once insulin therapy begins in type 1 diabetes treatment. Some individuals with insulin-dependent (type I) diabetes mellitus (IDDM), have even been known to control their weight by binging on food, but withholding their insulin. In the 1800s before insulin was created, someone with diabetes type 1 actually died of anorexia and complete wasting. Insulin is like the huge master lock that clasps in the body fat like a lock.

So now we know that the Harvard hospitals have it all wrong. It is not that insulin locks in body fat, and calories make fat. Carbohydrate makes the fat, and insulin delivers it and locks it in. Fat does not make you fat! Cheerios and oatmeal make you fat. Fat does not. Orange juice and grape juice make you fat. Fat does not. Challah and potato kugel make you fat. Fat does not!

Glycemic Index

Measured against Standard GI value Liquid Glucose (100 value) A comparison of insulin released compared to Liquid glucose

Glucose	100
Gatorade	78 +/-13
Cheerios	74
Oatmeal Quaker Oats	65
Coca Cola	63
Orange juice	53 +/-6
Chocolate Cadbury	49 +/- 6
Orange	48
Apple	40

Am J Clin Nutr January 1, 2002vol. 76 no. 1 5-56

See also back of book for complete
"Carbohydrate Count" and "Eat That, Not This" charts

Top Ten to Lose Ten

Cereal   Up to 40 grams per serving
Bread (whole grain or processed) and Rolls, bagels, muffins, etc. Up to 40 grams per serving
Orange juice (Grape juice, Apple juice, etc.) Up to 80 grams per glass
Crackers   Up to 40 grams per serving
Donuts   Up to 60 grams per donut
Cookies   Up to 40 grams per serving
Cake   Up to 60 grams per serving
Pizza   Up to 60 grams per serving
Carbonated soft drinks   Up to 60 grams per can
Chocolate Milk   Up to 40 grams per glass

3 The Heart of a Lonely Hunter

When one enters the Washington Zoo in America and enters the first exhibit hall, there is only to be found, a large floor to ceiling mirror. The sign reads: "The World's Most Dangerous Animal." Indeed, humans are the most feared, dangerous Carnivore on the planet. Think we are vegetarians or vegans? Think again? Humans are nothing like cows, sheep, horses, or deer. In Madagascar, 2,000 years ago, at least 15 species of primates went extinct after the arrival of humans. Humans not only hunted the primates but also burned and cut the forest, introducing domestic animals.[xxx] In Ecuador, Venezuela and Bolivia, around 40% of hunted animals are actually primates. Humans reign supreme in any habitat they inhabit. In neo-tropical countries, humans out-hunt pumas and jaguars. According to Michael Taube, we are Omnivores as described in his book, "The Omnivore's Dilemma." This sounds politically correct but humans are Carnivores. We have canine teeth, a large pancreas, the largest intestine of all animals per body length, and kill more animals than any other species each year. We are the least equipped to handle sugar from grain and fruit breakdown of any mammal. Unlike all other 2000 mammals on the planet, we cannot convert sugar to vitamin C, making us the most prone to diabetes and heart disease.

Primates and Humans are the only living creatures that cannot make Vitamin C of some 4000 mammals. Most other animals can synthesize vitamin C from glucose. Of 4,000 species of mammals, only humans and primates, along with a minor insect or fish, and the red-vented bulbul songbird, cannot synthesize vitamin C. This defect, arising through evolution, is considered an inborn error of metabolism. It may also explain why animals such as elephants, and other herbivores, are able to consume fruit without developing heart disease or obesity. Most animals produce 2-8 grams daily. Gorillas in the wild seek out about 4.5 grams of vitamin C a day. The Human requirement for Vitamin C is likely closer to this amount, than the government suggested RDA. Today, Vitamin C in high doses is being used to chelate or clear calcium deposits from human arteries. Early Vitamin C deficiency may explain on some level why some are more likely to develop arterial disease, as Vitamin C is essential to normal collagen, skin, and bone development. Animals other than primates may have reduced risk of heart disease as they convert sugar to Vitamin C.

In present day Paraguay, the Ache tribe hunts with their bare hands, proving beyond a doubt that humans are capable hunters, even without weapons or tools. They use only their bare hands or occasionally digging sticks. More than half of the game they capture are killed by hand.[xxxi] Humans match the bone breaking hyena in hunting prowess. African hunting dogs and lions can get returns two to ten times higher than humans can; however, humans have the intelligence to out-hunt any species with weapons.[xxxii] In India, humans regularly steal prey such as deer and wild boars from even the greatly feared and untrusted leopard.[xxxiii]

Humans are far more capable hunters than the two carnivorous primates, baboons and chimpanzees. Hunting returns for humans using traditional tools are from 10 to 200 times greater than for the largely insectivorous monkeys. All human hunter-gatherers get a much greater proportion of their daily food requirements from meat than any primate. For carnivorous baboons up to one fifth of the diet comes from insects and small animals. [xxxiv] A high fish, vegetable protein diet is healthier for us and the planet.

Until 200 years ago, Aborigines in Australia had a diet that was 50% protein, 40% fat, and 10% carbohydrate. By current criteria, all of such people were underweight, with a body mass index of 13 to 19.[xxxv] Studies of the Evenki reindeer herders in China indicate that they derive more than half their daily intake from meat. When comparing Evenki men with their U.S. peers, they are 20% leaner and have cholesterol levels that are 30% lower.[xxxvi]   73% of the worldwide hunter-gatherer societies derive more than half of the energy of their subsistence from animal foods.[xxxvii] They do not suffer any significant heart disease, or diabetes in any studies, until removed from their native countries or shipped in processed carbohydrates, grain staples, and Fanta beverages.

Lions and dolphins don't get heart disease from 50 pounds of meat and fish daily. Neither does the human carnivore. As wrong as Western indulgence for meat is today with low carbohydrate diets, this is not healthy, nor environmentally unfeasible It is merely spiritually degrading.

Young Mbuti Net Hunters consume as much as 86% of their diet from meat. Chippewayans Indians spent 98.6 % of their time obtaining meat and fish and only 1-4% of their foraging time gathering plant items.[xxxviii]   Fewer than 15% of hunter-gatherer societies throughout the world derive their subsistence from gathered plant foods.[xxxix] According to recent analysis, hunter-gatherers derive 40-60% of their energy from animal foods (meat, milk and other animal products). [xl] Even estimates of old world Europe before the Americas were settled show that approximately 60% of respective activities related to food were in hunting and fishing! [xli] Americans currently get only 12% of their diet in protein and close to 80% percent in grain and fruit. Once again, our intake of protein is currently less than a cow's consumption of protein from grass. Most reproductive disorders and aging are due to protein deficiency and carbohydrate overdose.

Carnivores have a significantly higher brain/body weight ratio than non-carnivores, as the human and the dolphin attest. [xlii] [xliii] 50-60% of brain solids are made out of fat. Fat intake is very important for pregnant and lactating women, and young children. The omega three fatty acids in fish oil EPA and DHA are essential to normal memory, learning, and mood. The natural source of these fats is actually found in seaweed. When fish consume the seaweed, they concentrate these essential oils in their fat tissues. High fish and seaweed consumption may explain one reason why Asia, Israel, and other neighboring sea nations have the highest measured IQ scores. Less than 1% of the omega three fat in flax seeds can get converted to EPA and DHA. A vegetarian diet does not have the same practical benefit to the brain and nervous system that fish oil does. Humans would have to eat thousands of flax seeds to have the same benefit as from fish.

We have explorations of Paleolithic diets. But we cannot figure out what we are today, hunter-gathering nomads, agrarian, or seafaring. We don't know whether we're carnivores, herbivores, granivores, frugivores, vegetarians or vegans.

High protein does not affect the kidneys. No studies to date have proved this conclusively. No fish goes into renal failure consuming 50 pounds of fish a day. And no lion succumbs to 12 pounds of meat a day. Japanese fisherman eating fish, tofu, and seaweed don't suffer renal failure. People with Diabetes and high blood sugar do. The pancreas of a dolphin is 300 grams. The human pancreas weighs 100 grams. Insectivores like the cow, and grass feeding ungulates have an almost non-existent pancreas.

Humans are Carnivores. Wildlife research supports that animals such as bears in the wild that are protein deficient have poor reproductive success, inability to conceive, and fewer surviving offspring. Primates who restrict their diet to fruit and insects have smaller brains, shorter life spans, and lower intelligence than carnivore primates. Those limited to largely an insect and vegetable diet have even smaller brains, less intelligence and shorter life spans. The more omega three in the diet, the better ones overall health and intelligence. Adding fish to one's diet is the key to long life, intelligence, and reproductive success. Most low carbohydrate plans such as Atkins and Sears recommend too much meat. Fish and legumes are a more wise method to get the protein we need. High consumption of fatty meat and chicken are linked to inflammation, cancer, high in hormones, pesticides, heavy metals. Anyone from PETA can tell you, kosher or not, most animals are mistreated. Small fish and legumes are a safer way to get one's protein. High meat intake is associated with increased Cancer risk and inflammatory disease. It does not however cause obesity or high cholesterol.

A majority of the planet today is entirely disconnected from the land. Only a tiny segment of the population is involved in farming. In contemporary times, our culture is not agricultural. It is sedentary. Between 300BCE and 500CE, the Ancient Physician and religious sage Maimonides, suggested that a normal healthy person consume only two meals a day and avoid excessive consumption of fruit or refined carbohydrates. Most of the corn and oats were fed to animals, and the majority of grapes were pressed for wine. The idea of juicing was completely foreign back then. Today, companies promote highly refined oat cereals and grape juice as a cure for heart disease and obesity. These refined foods today make up the leading cause of obesity. They are a blessing to cross a desert, or ocean, but in a sedentary society they are a ticket to high blood pressure and obesity.

High levels of exercise were fairly universal throughout history until the 1800s. A famous composer would walk 30 to 60 miles to hear a great musician. A painter might walk-25 miles a day, sketching as he walked. Abraham Lincoln was known to walk 15 miles to obtain a book he wanted to read.[xliv] Today, children watch television 2 hours a day. Many teenagers receive less than 20 minutes of physical education daily. The majority of adults are not regularly active.[xlv] We do not have as active a lifestyle as when society was largely agricultural, farming our own land and working in the fields. We don't work the fields from 6 am to 6 pm. We are not an agrarian society. Only 15% of Americans exercise on any given day. Americans spend 9 years of their lives watching TV, 151 hours a month, five hours a day.[xlvi] Agrarian diets high in grain and fruit are also not appropriate for a society that eats three large meals a day and snacks throughout the day. They are only appropriate for times when electricity did not exist, and activity levels were significant. We are neither hunters, gatherers, nor agrarian. Today, we are a largely service based, sedentary society.

There are many countries we could fly to for dietary wisdom. In the rainforests, we'd find chimpanzee and mongo nuts. In Okinawa, there are sashimi and seaweed. In Palm Beach, we'd see edamame and wheatgrass juice. However, we're only a plane ride away from finding out that most dinner tables look more similar than ever. A macrobiotic, human centered, eat local approach is not the answer. Not unless you are so myopic you think a 60% rice diet is the answer, along with local apples and pears in upstate Syracuse. Just as there is a global economy today, and international internet, there needs to be a global diet, a microbiotic one, rather than macrobiotic, an inspired approach that every nation can tap into for wisdom, rather than one constricted and limited to one's narrow own environment.

What we need now today is a microbiotic diet. Human life has never been static. Migrations have always been the norm in human existence. A macrobiotic diet keeps us standing still and looking at the man in the mirror. The answer for obesity is not found in Okinawa, Jerusalem, or the South Beach. That much has been proven, that the more we look at one country, the further we get from the Truth. Where can we turn for an honest answer today?

In Nature, there is neither such deception from business lobbies nor foreign powers from the outside. Nature offers the one last vestige of integrity where we can turn for honesty, Truth, Wisdom, and Understanding. Nature is constant and reliable. As Rabbi Akiva Tatz M.D. writes, "All of the Universe, from the planets to the atoms, all of biology, is reliable. ...No planet and no insect ever do what it is not supposed to do. Heaven and earth are reliable.

Only people are unreliable, that is the danger and price of free will."

We are told that if we never inherited the Torah to teach us ethics, we would have had to learn all our lessons from the animals. Today, we have to turn to Nature and Animals, because man has become untrustworthy and unreliable. Every medical study contradicts the other. Every diet says something different. Every month Huck and Tom are trying to repaint the same white fences on their block. A culture that breeds dishonesty and corruption cannot foster breakthroughs. The only safe haven today is nature, where even man cannot entirely impose himself. Everything in Nature follows its design. There is no such thing as an animal that doesn't have its role, sense of order and purpose. With thousands of hospitals and medical schools teaching essentially an entirely 100% fictitious story on cholesterol, obesity and heart disease, a person would have to be foolish to trust medical science for this information anymore. Most medical students hearing a lecture based on this book said that what convinced them the most were lessons on obesity from Nature and animals. The Truth has a way of breaking through all barriers. Medical students have almost built up an immunity to scientific data, because they are firsthand witnesses to the multitude of scientific studies that contradict each other daily, in the name of receiving a large grant from a pharmaceutical company. Medical students trust epidemiology and scientific studies about as much as the public trusts investment banks and law firms today.

Nothing in nature happens by coincidence. There are laws and rules in nature. Nothing is haphazard. The same can be said about each and every food we put into our body. The world of nature seems like a safe place to start for some refreshing honesty and some fresh perspective. Nature rarely sends mixed messages. There is little influence in the Animal Kingdom from pharmaceutical or medical industries. Rather than adapting the saying of the ancient physician and religious sage Maimonides, "everything in moderation," it would be wiser perhaps to adapt the saying of King Solomon, "To everything there is a season."

In the children's movie, "Ratatouille", a mouse becomes a famous Chef. When a food critic dines in the restaurant one evening, the young boy who owns the restaurant asks him what he would like for dinner. The critic responds, "You know what I'm craving? A little perspective. That's it. I'd like some fresh, clear, well seasoned perspective. Can you suggest a good wine to go with that?" Health books go for the bulls-eye, the big picture, the forest for the trees. But few seem to focus on the individual flowers, the wind in the background, the effect of the light on the tree, the colors that make up an individual fruit, or the crucial lesson from one of G-d's smallest creatures. Much like DaVinci used one invention as inspiration for another, and one seemingly unrelated technology led to another one, few medical scientists think today like engineers or artists. As the German Jewish poet Rainer Rilke once wrote:

You will not have to remain without a solution if you trust in Things that are like the ones my eyes are now resting upon. If you trust in Nature, in the small Things that hardly anyone sees and that can so suddenly become huge, immeasurable; if you have this love for what is humble and try very simply, as someone who serves, to win the confidence of what seems poor: then everything will become easier for you, more coherent and somehow more reconciling, not in your conscious mind perhaps, which stays behind, astonished, but in your innermost awareness, awakeness, and knowledge. ...Have patience with everything unresolved in your heart and to try to love the questions themselves as if they were locked rooms or books written in a very foreign language. Don't search for the answers, which could not be given to you now, because you would not be able to live them. And the point is, to live everything. Live the questions now. Perhaps then, someday far in the future, you will gradually, without even noticing it, live your way into the answer. xlvii

The birds and bees and many other animals have many powerful lessons for humans on how to eat properly. If we

34

consult a human on how to eat, we're led to a supermarket maze full of aisles and choices. Sometimes we have to start all over with the ABCs. Each of the four seasons offers a lesson. Sometimes we need the dark seasons to plant a seed and to plan for the future. Other seasons the rain comes and makes the seed grow. And when the sun then starts to shine, we will be rewarded with the patience that comes from the fruits of our labor. We need to look even to the wind, the sun, and even the water for novel insights and answers. For as Bob Dylan once wrote, "The Answer is Blowing in The Wind."

What we need first and foremost today is a Holistic diet that pays some attention to the spiritual health of our planet, and not just our stomach and our animal soul. Today, parts of the world are flooding while others are in drought. Similarly, half of the world struggles with poverty and hunger while obesity roars like a tidal wave through the rest. Our waists keep on growing. One in three Americans is obese. Our trees keep disappearing due to increased low carbohydrate diets and increased cattle production. Most of the diets in the last 10 years encourage a high animal protein "low glycemic" diet. This diet taken to its logical conclusion will literally wipe out our rainforests. "We do not live by bread alone." Weight loss is not a goal in itself. Spiritual and other concerns must guide our lives and our health. The ethics of our diet are rarely considered. It is difficult to be in touch with human nature, if we're completely out of touch with Mother Nature.

A high animal protein low carbohydrate diet may have made sense in the short term. But what if the rainforests were allowed to weigh in? Maybe we just might let the animals and trees have their say on the matter. Eating steak and red meat may be better for our arteries than table sugar, but it doesn't suggest good things in the next 100 years for our rain forests. Our environmental health and our physical health are interdependent. If we're going to increase our consumption of protein and lower our carbohydrate intake, we must also find new ways of conservation. Animals that are endangered need our protection. Our rainforests need preservation for our own long-term benefit.

While it is commonly believed that fat has the role of helping nature store fat, this is not the way Our Creator had in mind. Fruit and grain, are nature's answer for fat storage. Birds double their body fat when they fly south for the winter with the help of fruit alone. Bears double their body fat to hibernate with fruit, alone. And cows are fattened for market and industry with cereal grain and corn alone. Fruit assists animals in everything from starvation, the seasonal flight of birds, animal migrations, and hibernations, all conditions where weight gain is essential. They help humans through winter, food scarcity, and before electricity and cars, long distance migrations.

Why don't sharks get cancer, heart disease, or obesity? Nothing in the ocean eats grain and fruit. We humans wrongly promote these food groups as the most essential foods in our diet. Rather, they are the least essential for maintaining weight, well-being, happiness, and longevity. Fruit and grains may be natural but they were designed for a purpose, to help the body make and store fat and water. Natural and healthy are not always one and the same. We're not animals. And we shouldn't be eating like them. We say we want to eat naturally. But we don't even know ourselves. We can only truly know how to eat, with a perspective or comparison with Nature. Medical school is focused on human health and Veterinary and Wildlife Medicine is focused on Animal Health and these worlds need to finally be connected for their lessons. The reason why 1 in 2 is obese today has much to do with a lack of outpouring of wisdom from the other sciences into Medicine. We have so much to learn from Nature and Animals. To everything there is a season.

King Solomon once wrote that birds are the carriers of Truth. Every year, the sky of Israel fills with storks

36

returning from their winter migration. In Hebrew, the word for stork is "chasidah", which means kindness, because they take good care of their young. Out of the dark skies of winter, the stork is flying. "Be careful what you say, because birds are likely to carry your words."

To help humans in their long treks and nomadic voyages, nature invented a subtle food of choice, fruit. This allows plants to spread their seeds and humans and birds to carry them along for the ride. There is a time to plant seeds and a time to harvest. There is a time to stand still and a time to fly.

During the year, birds eat insects, seeds, worms, and plants. Only a small handful of birds are fruit eaters, fewer than 10% of all birds. During the fall, they make a dramatic switch, a 180 degree turn to eating fruit. This fruit enables them to generate immense obesity for wintertime flights to warmer regions of the world. The entire length of the year, they consume sources of protein and fat. They do this for good health and to give birth to healthy young. One short month of the year, they appear to follow their nose to fruit.

Over 90% of birds are insectivores.[xlviii] Before migration, birds such as Northern Water thrush, Shorebirds, and Arctic land birds shift their diet to nearly one hundred percent fruit. They will eat fruit during this time even though many insect species (Orthoptera, Deptera, and Arachnida) are widely abundant until early October.[xlix] Gray Cat-birds, Yellow-rumped Warblers, (Evans 1966, Herrera 1984, Bairlein 1990, Izhakki 1989), (Parrish 1997, 2000) and Songbirds rely solely on fruit in the fall, even though many protein sources are also still available to them. This isn't a choice of availability but one of necessity. Because only sugar can create body fat, not protein or fat necessary for long flights.[l,li,lii] Those who fail to find fruit may not survive the journey.[liii] Birds have enormously fast metabolisms and often eat 10% of their body weight of insect protein.[liv] Over half the birds in the world make non-stop flights of up to 3,600 to 22,000 miles. Some 300 to 500 species of birds in North America partake in winter migration.[lv lvi] The Ducks marshes are filled with ice. Insect eaters travel to the Gulf States or Tropics. An Arctic Tern flies 22,000 miles to her final destination[lvii] This flight requires that they generate sufficient body fat beforehand to allow them to survive the long trip. Long flights require not only enormous endurance but massive obesity.[lviii]

Garden Warblers eat so much fruit that they are named "The Fig eater ("Beccafico"). A monarch butterfly doubles its body weight on fruit nectar before its winter flight.[lix] They say the wind behind a butterfly in Los Angeles; can power a tidal wave across the world. Most butterflies migrate relatively short distances (Painted Ladies, Red Admirals, and Buckeyes), but a few, such as Monarchs, migrate thousands of miles.[lx] Fruit-eating species of birds are more successful in acquiring further body mass during flight stopovers to refuel on more fruit for their journey.[lxi] Some birds eat so much fruit and cereal fed by humans, that they eventually lose their power of flight. Muscovy ducks are crammed with corn feed down their throats, for two to three weeks to fatten their livers to make" foie gras."[lxii] Each duck is fed the equivalent of over nearly 40 pounds of pasta to make foie gras.

When breeding season comes in the spring, birds switch back to their normal diet, from nectar, fruit, and seeds to a largely protein diet, aquatic insects. They feed their offspring largely insects in summer and even shellfish in the winter. They only feed their young berries to prepare for migration in the fall.

Hummingbirds feed on sugar-rich nectars. Unlike humans, a capacity to convert sugar to vitamin C prevents them from developing obesity or heart disease. Most other fruit-eating birds are unable to digest sucrose and prefer fructose nectars.[lxiii] A hummingbird's metabolism is 10

38

times faster than an elite athlete's is. Her wings beat 50 times a second, her heartbeats 1,260 a minute and she inhales 250 breaths in one minute.[lxiv] To recover, she enters a state of deep sleep. [lxv] [lxvi]

A baby bird isn't made out of sugar. Neither are we. A baby isn't made out of carbohydrate. But we often eat like we are. Virtually nothing in our body is made out of sugar other than our body fat. A healthy diet year-round is a fertility diet. If baby-making is your goal, this is a valuable lesson. A lesson from birds for humans who want healthy children and fertile parents is, "Follow your nose!" This may be the difference between flying like a butterfly and being stung like a bee. Perhaps the simple "birds and the bees" of nutrition may be, "If it isn't green and it doesn't move quickly, eat of it sparingly.

When we wander away from Nature and try to fight it, it is always Nature who wins. When we wander off the path the bear helps us get back on track. If we continue to eat junk food, and smoke, it is written, a small hole in the body produces a large hole in the soul. And in the end, disease can overtake a person like a bear. The farmers have an expression, "one day off sets a person back two days." When you're eating well and maintaining good health habits, this is even more encouragement to keep up these positive habits. The bear may slumber through the winter but the rest of the year, he is a hunter, chasing fish and game. The bear is not one to stand over the river. He's active, engaged, and knows how to get his hands dirty. To find what he's looking for, he has to look beneath the surface of the water. Without diets, it is the same way, as long as we are at least in the water, doing the swimming, we are in good shape. If we get distracted by all the allure of what crass commercialism promises us, quick fixes for obesity, where all you have to do is eat what you want, and take a quick pill, come on, does anyone really believe this. To lose weight, you have to get your hands wet. There's no easy answer. And no free lunch.

As the temperature is beginning to fall, the little bear is lined up right behind the bluebird at the berry bushes. The food that helps a bear pack on three hundred pounds in the winter is fruit. The saying goes, "an apple a day keeps the doctor away." For the bear, the apple tree means weight gain. The food that helps a bear become more than just the average bear is fruit, mostly berries. Whether the porridge is too hot or cold, the bear will take as many carbohydrates as offered to hibernate.

In the course of an autumn day, a bear will feast on tens of thousands of berries. A bear will go on feeding frenzies. A binge might include 10,000 grapes in a day, a vineyard. A fruit diet in the fall helps a bear accumulate up to 212 pounds of fat for hibernation. (Bears. Wood, Daniel. Whitecap Books. Vancouver, Canada. 1995.)[lxvii] The greatest weight of an American brown bear ever measured was 803 lbs. back in 1885 in Stevens Point, Wisconsin.[lxviii] If someone is trying out for a beauty show, going on an all fruit or "raw fruit" diet, or even worse, fruit juicing, is not the answer. Fruit might be natural. But if you're not a bird or a bear, it is the recipe to diabetes. Bears also convert fruit sugar to Vitamin C, unlike humans, which is why they don't get diabetes.

All types of berry will do for a bear--- blackberries, dewberries, salmon berries, crow berries, huckleberries, mountain ash berries, and bear berries. Fruit forms more than 90% of their diet in the fall.[lxix lxx lxxi lxxii lxxiii lxxiv lxxv] Bears also have a well-known fondness for honey. When a bear comes upon a wild bee tree, it eats the honey, wax, and bees all together. An insect's sting does not affect the bear's mouth and bears are found with quarts of yellow jackets in their stomachs.[lxxvi lxxvii]

A bear's main diet during the year consists of fish, insects and other animals. Grizzlies mostly hunt ungulate, elk, bison, and moose.[lxxviii lxxix] In Yellowstone, meat constitutes nearly 80% of the annual diet for a Grizzly in the spring. In Tibet, bears consume plateau pika, wild yaks, and antelopes. Pine nuts or acorns may also be chewed in the fall, but fruit is the primary component of the diet in the fall. [lxxx] Vegetation is only a small part of the diet in all seasons.[lxxxi lxxxii lxxxiii] In Colombia, Bolivia, and Spain, bears prey on cattle farms and.[lxxxiv] in Sweden, ants are an important year round source of protein.[lxxxv] .

Their appetite for berries in autumn is equally matched by their fierceness for fish and meat, the rest of the year. In the summertime, the salmon start to run.[lxxxvi] To stay light on their feet while salmon hunting in the spring, fish and sea vegetation is the food of choice. [lxxxvii] Bears can survive without salmon, but tend to be smaller in height and have fewer children. The size of non-salmon eating bear populations are one fiftieth the size of salmon-feeding populations.[lxxxviii lxxxix]

Polar bears are the largest bear in the world, up to 8 feet tall. They are found mostly in Greenland, Norway, and Alaska.[xc] They feed on large fish, seals, and walrus. When a bear eats a seal it gorges itself upon the blubber, but disregards the muscle, which they leave for foxes.[xci xcii] Coastal bears such as those found in Alaska feed on a variety of fish, barnacles, and sea vegetation.

Our health authorities say, "six servings of fruit a day." This sounds more like a bear preparing for hibernation! For humans, the result of excess consumption of fruit leads to just this--- an early hibernation under the apple trees. If one wants to be 800 pounds--- (if one truly wants to double their body fat), a patch of berries or a honey jar is a sure ticket. The word natural today has become synonymous with "healthy", and this couldn't be further from the Truth. As the bear illustrates, a hand too often in the honey jar is likely to be stung. For good health, numerous and healthful offspring, protein, fats and vegetables are your wise year-round choices. In the Talmud, the word bear, "dov", means wanderer. When we become complacent, or let our standards of spiritual and physical health fall, it is said, the bear comes to awaken us from our slumber.[xciii xciv] By now hopefully you are getting the point that body fat is made from sugar, and not from fat. For more support, there are valuable lessons from animals being fed on the farm to fatten them. There is further proof for us being a Carnivore from the Cat, the cow, and the elephant. And proof that fat is good for the brain, from the monkey. But if you are convinced, then maybe proceed now to read the section on heart disease, where you will learn how sugar, not cholesterol is the cause of all arterial disease, from blindness, renal disease, sexual dysfunction, and brain disease. For those fascinated by the animals, as most of my medical student friends, and professors, and those in the health field, it is the animal information that might be most interesting and relevant. It will enhance your perspective on disease greatly. For those with little knowledge of human medicine or health, the section on the heart or Cancer prevention, as well as the 10 spiritual steps would be recommended reading. Books like "Good Calories Bad Calories" have made hundreds of pages of medical studies, the legal case against carbohydrates, and disproving cholesterol. But they haven't done a good job because people are skeptical now of Medicine and scientists with dishonest science. Animals are a clear, refreshing, and honest perspective. But Truth be told, sometimes we don't need 100 pages of scientific studies to convince us. For me, reading about the cow, was what gave me the final proof that we do not get fat from fat. 1000 studies couldn't convince me otherwise. It's not about quantity of information, but quality, and most books today are simply rehashing "The Zone" diet. The real gold is to be found in veterinary circles for obesity. The Torah wasn't given at the tallest mountain in Israel, but the smallest, and most humble. Likewise, many of our important lessons in life are found from the humble, small places we ignore.

Cereal is still touted as the breakfast of champions. It's whole grain, so it has to be natural and good, people say.

For farm animals, cereal feed is the main method of fattening animals for human consumption.

We feed zoo animals cereal and we fatten cattle with cereal for beef production. We offer it to horses for animal feed and to birds in the park. In the wild, these animals graze on grass, not grain. What sugar they do consume gets converted to vitamin C, unlike in humans. The rest goes to pack on body fat.

Nothing in the ocean eats cereal and fruit, including sea mammals such as dolphins, sea lions and porpoises. However, the ungulates (cows, sheep, and elephants) with multiple stomachs do not eat cereal due to its low vitamin content. They feed on grass, plants, herbs, and sprouting vegetables. Cereal for them is junk food. They eat it out of desperation. No cereal makes the top twenty of vitamins and minerals. Cows eat wheat grass, not wheat.

From spring to winter, Cows feed on green pasture. Cattle farmers confine them to feedlot grains to fatten them for market. The industrial name for this process is "finishing." It takes one-third the time to "finish" a cow on grain than it would on grass. Grains add marbling and fat to the cow but contribute little else.[xcv] Carbohydrate feeding of cattle is more economical and speeds up their fat gain. It also helps keep dairy cows producing milk 365 days a year. The more grain a cow is fed, the more marbled they become.[xcvi] Dairy farming of cows ensures the meat is also full of added hormones and may be the leading cause of prostate Cancer, Japanese research shows. It is also cruel to the cow, which normally does not milk 365 days a year.

In the United States, corn maize is the most commonly used.[xcvii xcviii xcix] Cows everywhere across the world, in Australia, Japan, and Korea are all fattened with grain.[c] In the Middle East and Europe, barley and soy meal are used.[ci] Cows in Canada are finished on cereal and barley grain. Bulls are fattened industrially on finishing diets of either cereals or sugar beets. In Yugoslavia, corn is the preferred agent of obesity.[cii] In the most common lamb-finishing system in Spain, feedlot lambs feed on all barley diets until they their finished weights. [ciii] It requires approximately 200–260 days from weaning to finishing to produce highly marbled or grade 'A' beef with live weights ranging between 450 and 600 kg.[civ]

Grass is alone a good source of protein (7-10%). It is one of nature's perfect foods. It has many times the vitamins and minerals of garden vegetables.[cv] Cows possess multiple stomachs to digest this grass. The cow, camel, elephant, giraffe, deer, sheep, buffalo, and antelope are called "ruminants."[cvi] Giraffe consume the least grass of browsers and buffalo the most. All members of the ungulate family are actually insectivores, not vegetarians. [cvii] Pigs, peccaries, and hippos, have more varied diets that includes small animals.[cviii] In nature, there is no true vegetarian larger than the size of a mouse. Even the rarely moving koala which sits in a tree eating leaves all day, regularly consumes insects on any foliage. Most cattle farms however, feed their cows and lambs with diets entirely absent of grass and forage.[cix] One of the side effects of extensive grain feeding is impaired reproductive functioning. Cows, like the birds and the bears, cannot reproduce successfully without sufficient protein from grass and insects.[cx] Grain feeding also causes acidosis, microbial overgrowth, and indigestion.[cxi] A cow's stomach is not suited for concentrated cereal starch. They will lick their own coats and other cows' in order to increase the fiber in their diet. The large amounts of hair eventually go on to cause abscesses, or infections in their rumen (stomach).[cxii] Once upon a time, cattle were wild throughout the world. Grass-fed cows are usually thin, fit, and can run. But because they've been turned into industrial strength grain feeders, today they can barely even move.

So which makes a cow more obese? Cereal is animal food. It's meant to fatten cows for market, a process aptly called finishing. It is not consumed by any of the 2000 other

44

mammals on the planet. Is there any cereal in the ocean? Dolphins, porpoises and sea lions don't watch breakfast cereal commercials. Kids have to think outside the box, and out of the bowl. In general, if it doesn't have to be refrigerated, leave it outside the kitchen. Breakfast cereal, because of its daily use, is the most dangerous food in the world. Instead of suing McDonalds for fried fish sandwiches, our Congress should be regulating Cereal, cookie, and cake producers. Understand this.

There is no support in nature that carnivores in the wild are obese on high protein, high fat diets. More often, the more herbivorous and frugivorous land animals are highest in body fat. Humans actually have more in common with carnivores than herbivores.[cxiii]

Elephants eat 16-17 hours a day. [cxiv] When elephants have been feeding in a certain area for weeks the area takes years to become fertile again.[cxv] The African elephant is the largest living land animal. It weighs almost 6 tons. An elephant's diet consists of about one third grass. [cxvi] They also have a fondness for ants and termites. Their favorite is the elephant tree.[cxvii cxviii] Because their diet is not nutrient dense, they must consume a great deal more food than carnivores. Carnivores and humans need one to three high nutrient meals a day. Despite calls for humans to eat five small meals a day, humans are not meant to be grazers or browsers, eating all day long like an elephant.[cxix cxx cxxi]

We humans are Carnivores, not vegetarians, not herbivores, and not insectivores. Despite books that may have you convinced, that we are "omnivores", this is an inaccurate and vague concept, as misleading as the word "calorie". We humans are omnivores out of ignorance, not by choice. We cannot digest grass so we are not technically herbivores. We neither spend our time browsing nor grazing. We do not employ bacterial hind-gut fermentation, such as elephants and hippos. Elephants are known as hind-gut fermenters. Their guts house large numbers of bacteria and protozoa that help digest cellulose in plants. We are not ruminators and do not regurgitate grass like the cow. In terms of tooth structure, humans share more similarity with carnivores. We have canines and ridge molars not flat teeth of herbivores or insectivores. [cxxii] Ruminant herbivores such as sheep, deer, and buffalo have no canines. They have no teeth on the front of their upper jaw at whatsoever. We humans have multi-ridged molars as opposed to flat molars found in ungulates with two sets of incisors on top and bottom. We use canines to sever bones of mammalian prey and for shearing flesh from bone, not to chew grass or plants. Humans also chew their food in vertical motions rather than rotary motions as herbivores. [cxxiii] And our pancreas size for our body weight suggests we were meant to eat and digest meat. Grass has so much more digestive enzymes so a goat or cow does not need a large pancreas. An herbivore's intestines are always full. Yet humans like other carnivores usually empty their stomachs in 3-4 hours. Herbivores have long and bulky digestive tracts while carnivores and humans have short and simple digestive tracts. The digestive system of elephants measures around 27.5 meters compared to 7 meters for humans. Not only this, but based on our body size, we have the shortest intestine: body size ratio. It's not just the length therefore which helps classify us as a carnivore. Plant matter requires long digestive tracts to digest. Animal matter, both vertebrate and invertebrate, requires a simpler digestive tract. [cxxiv] The digestibility of meat is also higher than grains or beans. Meat, dairy, and eggs are 94-97% digestible. Grains and beans are "only" 78-85% digestible. [cxxv] We humans are on the top of the food chain, greater killers than any other species. Our brain is the most complex, and we are smarter than any other Carnivore such as dolphins, primates, or sea lions and porpoises. Subcutaneous fat is unique to humans, primates, walruses, sea cows, babirusas, whales, and dolphins, all Carnivores and none vegetarian. All animals eat insects and are insectivores, even the koala.

Length of digestive system

Dog	7 m
Humans	7 m
Pony	13.1 m
Zebra	17.2 m
Elephant	27.5 m
Indian Rhino	31.1 m
Horse	31.3 m
Cow	60 m

Are there animals that survive without grain and fruit?
There is such an animal! This would clearly then support
than fruit and cereal grain are not essential for a living
animal. Cats have no carbohydrate in their natural diet at
all. Most cat food is 90% carbohydrate, to save money for
the food companies. They fatten cats, the same way
farmers fatten cattle. The diet of the lion, leopard, cheetah,
African wild dog, and hyena are entirely meat-based,
coming 100% from animals.[cxxvi] [cxxvii]

Some Carnivores are meat specialists such as cats, seals and
dolphins. Some are bone crackers such as hyenas, and
others have more varied diets which include vegetables and
legumes, seeds, and nuts, such as coyotes, dogs, bears,
humans, and primates. [cxxviii]

The most common food of foxes includes mammals (92%)
and birds with a small percentage of their diet coming from
plants. They rarely, like a cat, will touch fruit! A fox will
eat fruit only as a supplementary food resource and as
mammal populations decrease. In Italy, a group of wolves
that snuck into a farm consumed 200 sheep. (Now that's a
snack!) Wild dogs found in Africa mainly prey on
antelopes. Cape hunting dogs are extremely fast and can
even outrun foxes and coyotes.[cxxix] Seals, dolphins, and
other sea mammals survive on fish.[cxxx] How is this? The
reason there is no absolute requirement for carbohydrate in
the diet is because protein can be broken down into
sugar.[cxxxi] Humans are capable of converting as much as

half of their protein into glucose.[cxxxii]   A dog or a fox makes more than half of its blood glucose from dietary protein.[cxxxiii]   We have to question the importance of fruits and grains in our diet above vegetables in the USDA food recommendations. After all, if cats and all marine life do not rely on fruits and grains in their diet, how essential are they outside of vitamin C, found in larger amounts in vegetables than fruits anyways.

Just as for cows, dogs, and dolphin, there is no essential carbohydrate in the human or animal diet. There are essential fatty acids. There are essential amino acids, but no "essential" carbohydrate. There is no such thing as a "carbohydrate free" protein diet as protein digestion provides all the essential glucose required for life.   A cow survives on a grass diet and insects. Birds eat primarily insects and worms. Dolphins, penguins, and pelicans feed almost exclusively on fish. The dog is a carnivore and cats cannot digest fruit, or fructose, at all.

Walking down the supermarket aisle shopping for your dog or cat isn't much different than the supermarket in general. The shelves are usually nothing but carbohydrate. It is as though dog food manufacturers and cereal companies have the same goals, to fatten us all.   Most dog foods are 80% starch. Although they haven't invented sugar coated dog food, it makes one wonder that we feed our children sometimes not much better than we feed our pets. In newborn dogs, high carbohydrate dog food is the major cause of overweight puppies.[cxxxiv]   Although domestic cats retain an ability to hunt better than pet dogs, today's high carbohydrate cat foods have led to more than a quarter of domestic cats being overweight. Forty percent of cats seen in one clinic in Denmark are overweight or obese.[cxxxv]   We do not knowingly feed our pets carbohydrate, because of our concern for diabetes, blindness, and obesity. Unfortunately, carbohydrate still forms the staple of our human diet.

Unlike dogs, cats are pure carnivores and cannot eat fruit.[cxxxvi][cxxxvii] The taste buds of cats are completely insensitive to sugar.[cxxxviii] They also cannot synthesize Vitamin A or arachidonic acid. When cats are fed vegetarian diets which are deficient in arachidonic acid they develop respiratory infections and loss of oestrus or ability to ovulate.[cxxxix][cxl] Even with all meat diets, Carnivores, including cats, lions, tigers, owls, and fox all have the higher blood sugar than herbivores.[cxli] Plasma glucose levels are actually higher in dogs fed all meat diets than high carbohydrate diets. Herbivores such as horses, sheep, cattle, and rats have the lowest blood sugar levels when fasting.[cxlii] Caribou, reindeer, and camels maintain moderate glucose levels. [cxliii]

Would cats, dogs, bears, and members of the carnivore family be better off eating whole grain breads and cereals or fruit or chewing on hot dogs, hamburgers, and cheese? First, without protein, they will not reproduce. Second, these animals develop diabetes in a matter of weeks on bread, cereal, and fruit. Third, like we humans, they rely on two to three high quality, meaning high protein and fat meals a day, for normal functioning. Other carnivores, such as Cats typically feed two to three times a day. Dogs, who hunt in packs, can rely on one big meal. This suggests that humans are not grazers or browsers, but hunters, like cats and dogs. We need to eat once to three times a day, like other carnivores.

Wild cats are the human equivalent of long distance runners and short distance sprinters. They are the fastest runners on the planet. Some believe that fat is dangerous when compared with sugar. Does the natural food of a carnivore such as a cat, an exclusive meat diet, really harm their arteries? A Bengal Tiger can consume 50 pounds of meat in one meal.[cxliv][cxlv] Leopards are among the strongest predators of humans and are believed to be one of the major selective factors in the evolution of humans and primates. The ability of large cats to prey on primates may have been what caused primates to develop and manipulate weapons out of trees and rocks and later craft more sophisticated methods to ward off attacks. [cxlvi]

Robert Atkins and Richard Bernstein, the low carbohydrate camp, are closer to the Truth than the low insulin diet camp led by Barry Sears. They're both wrong. There's no requirement for carbohydrate. Why? There is no requirement for sugar for a living organism. All sea mammals break down protein to provide sugar for red blood cells, the only part of the body that requires it. So there is no carbohydrate required for life. Only essential amino acids and essential fatty acids. Our brain uses any source of fuel, not just glucose. The brain may be the fuel hog of the body. However, it can run even preferentially on fat (ketones), the recommendation for most with seizure or brain disease. High blood sugar is known to cause neuropathy, including eye movement, heartbeat, brain function, and peripheral neuropathy. Too much sugar is not good for the brain.

Primates such as monkeys share the most similar physical and physiological characteristics with humans. Subcutaneous fat is unique to humans, primates, walruses, sea cows, babirusas, whales, and dolphins.[cxlvii] This is further support that we are Carnivores. All these mammals are carnivores.

All apes, including chimpanzees, orangutans, gorillas, gibbons, and the siamang, eat insects. [cxlviii cxlix cl cli clii cliii] Apes prefer meat to all other foods. [cliv clv clvi clvii] Baboons can hunt medium size antelopes. They have the largest brains of any primate after humans.[clviii] Chimpanzees will also kill and eat animals, mostly other primates. Primates account for 62-100% of chimpanzee prey at study sights in West and East Africa.[clix] Leopards and other primates are the only feared predators in eastern and southern African savannah. [clx] Chimpanzees are the most capable in avoiding predation.[clxi clxii clxiii]

Chimpanzees resemble humans more than gorillas and share 98.6% of the same DNA with humans. They can show affection, altruism, and aggression. They will hunt in packs and they share food.[clxiv][clxv][clxvi][clxvii][clxviii] Chimpanzees are the most dexterous mammals, along with otters and raccoons. They are able to craft weapons for hunting, defense, and to dig up insects underground. Unlike humans, Chimpanzees have at most three pounds of body fat.[clxix] This may have to do with their constant movement and the necessity of hunting. Or they simply don't consume grains and grain products like humans.

The most important attribute associated with intelligence and long lifespan in primates is the level of fat consumption. Across all primates, species with the larger brains dine on higher fat foods.[clxx] Those with the shortest lives and smallest brains are leaf-eating colobines.[clxxi] Primates with medium size brains live on insects. [clxxii] And Old world monkeys with the longest life spans are those with the largest brains and most meat in the diet, mandrills and baboons. Gibbons and orangutans consume more fruit than chimpanzees and live a shorter lifespan.[clxxiii]

Primates typically consume protein sources such as honey, vertebrates, invertebrates and tree proteins. None are considered vegetarians. This is the strongest argument yet, that humans were not supposed to be vegans or vegetarians. Some Colobines and gorillas are able to consume leaves similar to ungulates. They have large numbers of microbes which assist in fermentation and a 4 chambered stomach like the cow.[clxxiv][clxxv] . The only rare instance of an extreme folivore, or leaf eater in nature, is the Koala, a type of bear. It weighs just 6 kg and has an enormous intestine of almost 2 meters for its small size. They consume up to 1.5 kg of leaves and insects, which they digest over a period of days. They move around only 1 percent of the time as their diet is so energy poor.[clxxvi]

4 Of Mice and Men—Toxic Medicine

In the 1980s, two scientists won an award for the discovery of a disease called familial hypercholesterolemia, a 1 in 2 million disorder that produces an instant heart attack. The disorder is as rare as a leopard striking someone dead in the heart of a Manhattan cross-street. But this didn't stop the science academia from enthroning it for life, "the cause" of a heart attack. To set the record straight, it is the rarest cause of a heart attack, however lethal. A lie well told is immortal.

Diabetes Type II is the leading statistic cause of blindness, kidney disease, dialysis, impotence, and limb amputation. We're standing on a river and refusing to notice. Cardiologists take to heart only the lessons of a rare 1 in 2 million disorder, a paper tiger. Diabetes is found in more than 1 in 3 patients undergoing heart surgery.[clxxvii] High blood sugar is the leading cause today of a heart attack, not high cholesterol, despite widespread belief.[clxxviii] [clxxix] [clxxx] And—if you do believe cholesterol plays a role in heart disease outside this rare disorder (which it does not), be aware that the same pathway for making fat in the fat cell applies to the liver. This is why over 20 studies now show that fat in the blood rises (Triglycerides) with diabetes, and decreases as the percent of fat rises, and carbohydrate lowers. These studies can be found on any medical database and are even found in a few low carbohydrate diet books. But it goes beyond this. Fat doesn't cause heart disease. It is diabetes, and high blood sugar. The fat is called a confounding error. It appears high, so it is associated with a rise in heart disease. But the only reason it is high, is because the sugar is high, which is the real culprit in the oxidation process of the artery. Cholesterol being high doesn't mean it is the culprit. Cholesterol is the innocent bystander.

From 1935 to 1996, Diabetes Type II rose nearly seven-fold. The global figures are predicted to rise 46% from 150 million cases in 2000 to 221 million by 2010. [clxxxi] Since

1990, the number of adults diagnosed with diabetes has more than doubled. The incidence in Japan doubled in teenagers from 1985 to 1996.[clxxxii]

By comparison, let's look at an insignificant disease on the radar, familial hypercholesterolemia. The risk of full blown familial hypercholesteremia (FH) is only one in 2 million.[clxxxiii] FH is a disease where the body has no receptors to remove cholesterol from the blood, leading to, well, essentially, suffocation, and a stream of lard in the arteries. The risk of inheriting one gene for this rare disorder is one in 500.[clxxxiv] If someone came into a medical clinic with asthma, and the doctor proclaims to the patient, "You have cystic fibrosis." we'd know something was very wrong. But this is just what is happening with heart disease. The disease is as rare as being killed by a cheetah in Manhattan but Harvard area doctors made it the most common cause of a heart attack over fifty years ago.

Glucose and fructose attach themselves to every artery. When sugar glues itself to retinal arteries it leads to blindness. When it caramelizes arteries in the heart this leads to a heart attack. When it binds and sugar coats arteries in the kidneys it leads to kidney failure. When it binds to arteries in the brain, dementia and cranial neuropathy ensue. When small arteries in the hands and lower limbs get affected in advanced disease, limb amputation is the result. A crank cannot pass caramel and glue through a body forever. Passing glue through an engine, and your body's cells, won't last forever before the engine gets stuck.

Everything you know you learned in kindergarten. In school, we teach children how to make glue by mixing cornstarch and water. Fats, also known as lipids, run along our arteries like hot oil running smoothly across an engine. Glucose, on the other hand, is like sludge in a motor. The quickest way to make glue is by using sugar, not fat. Glucose forms a caramel-like substance that glues itself to every fat and protein in the body. Meat may spoil and seeds may mold, but sugar, like fruit, rots, from the inside out. The process by which sugar damages arteries is called "glycosylation". Glycosylation of red blood cells, when sugar binds on to red blood cells, impairs the ability to carry oxygen, and is the cardinal sign of high blood sugar. When sugar (carbohydrate) coats white blood cells immunity is reduced by 50%. When they coat neutrophils which fight bacteria, it is harder to fight infections, which happens in diabetes, for this reason and because of reduced oxygen and blood flow with the arterial disease sugar causes. When sugar coats natural killer cells which fight viruses and tumor cells, this can lead to increased colds and even Cancer. Think sugar only binds red and white blood cells? It is not inconceivable that even sperm may be subject to fructosylation, leading to infertility. The same process that eventually leads to diabetic calcification (Monk berg's calcification), is glycosylation. Arteries bound by glucose, are eventually attacked by macrophages and other immune cells, leading to calcium release from arterial cells, blocked arteries, heart attacks, and strokes.[clxxxv]

Again, high blood sugar is the leading cause of blindness, end-stage renal failure, non-traumatic limb amputations, sexual dysfunction, neuropathy, and cardiovascular mortality. Sound a lot like widespread arterial disease?[clxxxvi] [clxxxvii] Diabetic nephropathy is the leading cause of end-stage renal disease in the United States.[clxxxviii] No fisherman ever checks into the doctor's office and says, Doc, I'm eating too much fish and tofu, my kidneys are failing. But I have seen thirty year olds with legs amputated from high blood sugar. This is because sugar entering the network of fat and protein creates literal caramel and glue. Humans are not bagels. We're made of protein and fat, like animals. And when you stir sugar into fat, you make caramel and glue. When you stir fat into a pan with hot oil, it doesn't stick. Stir sugar into oil, and you'll be cleaning that pan for hours. In the body, it's the same. Because diabetes is defined as high blood sugar, which results from high carbohydrate intake, carbohydrate, not fat consumption, is the most important statistical predictor of a heart attack.

Not convinced? A bottle nose dolphin eats 50 pounds of fish daily, 5% of its 1000 pound weight, without suffering ill-health. A lion eats between 12 to 15 pounds of meat a day, 2% of their 600 pound body weight. Some diets for a small common house cat recommend over 4 pounds of meat a day. The pancreas of a dolphin is 300 grams. The human pancreas weighs 100 grams. Does any shark eating 50 pounds of fish in the water, 20 pounds of it fat, keel over every day in the ocean? Are scores of lions turning over in the jungle from 50 pounds of meat each day? Fat doesn't cause a heart attack. Whether glue is poured quickly or slowly over an artery, it sticks, whether the person is a professional sprinter, marathon runner, or professional couch potato. Glue sticks regardless of how fast the engine is working. And so it is not than lions or dolphins don't suffer heart disease eating fifty pounds of meat and fish daily because they're exercising, but because they don't eat carbohydrates. And because fat doesn't cause heart disease.

Statistics on carbohydrates and their influence on disease states:

Leading cause of heart attack: Diabetes type II (high blood sugar)
Current percent of obese women in America: 50%
Individuals with Diabetes Type II who are obese: greater than   90%
Americans with Diabetes type II: 16%
Americans with Insulin resistance (producing too much insulin):   25%
Americans who are Glucose intolerant: 10%

The Statistics on cholesterol:

Homozygous familial hypercholesteremia:
ONLY 1 in 1 million individuals!
(the one that produces a heart attack)

Heterozygous familial hypercholesteremia:
1 in 500 individuals

Leading cause of:

	Sugar	Cholesterol
Diabetes	Yes	No
Blindness	Yes	No
Renal failure	Yes	No
Non-trauma Limb amputation	Yes	No
Sexual dysfunction	Yes	No
Heart Attack	Yes	No
Obesity	Yes	No

Denmark Study on deaths per 100,000

Year	Deaths	Sugar Intake Per Person / Year
1880	1.8	13.5 kg.
1911	8.0	37.6 kg.
1934	19.1	51.3 kg.
1955	34.3	74.7 kg.
1975	78.6	81.8 kg.

http://befreetech.com/sugar_sweet_poison.html

No pure carnivore like the lion or tiger eats grain or fruit. And no insectivores like cows, elephants, goats, sheep, and etc.eat grain or fruit. Making humans quite literally the most stupid animal on the planet, when it comes to Nutrition. Nothing they teach at Harvard Medical School will help you here. You cannot rely on a human model today because in China, there are cookies and cereals from all over the world. Every country today is a miniature copy of every other, and with airplanes, food from one country finds itself in every other. Chinese restaurants and Japanese restaurants are found all over the world. Looking at the Chinese, the Japanese or the Italians for answers on heart disease is like looking at ourselves in the mirror.

It is said that the eyes are the windows to the soul. If one's eyes are healthy, one's heart is all the more likely to be healthy as well. This is why vision loss and impotence are such potent signs of impending heart disease. Those with high carbohydrate diets are 40% more likely to suffer from macular degeneration of the eye.[clxxxix] Eye disease is nothing more than an impending sign of heart disease, just like cataracts and glaucoma in the eye. The eyes are truly more than windows to the soul. Early diagnosis of retinal disease can be a lifesaver. Among humans, small hunter-gatherer tribes typically have dental cavities. There was a clear increase in gum disease and dental cavities associated with the rise of agriculture in Native Americans and Egypt. The much higher cavity rates of the last two centuries are associated with increases in grains and fruits in the diet. This decay is not limited to teeth, but also found on an arterial level. Being thin is no immunity to heart disease.

Diabetes predisposes someone to a doubled risk of heart disease. The risk of diabetes goes up almost 20% with each glass of orange juice a day, according to one study, as much as for a glass of coca cola. Orange juices, and breakfast cereal, because of their vast consumption, are the leading cause of heart disease, as great as a soda! An Italian study in the Archives of Internal Medicine followed nearly 48,000 adults including about 32,500 women from 2002 to determine which diets were most likely to lead to heart disease. In the study, the female participants who consumed the most carbohydrates had about twice the risk of heart disease. Greater than 70% of mortality in diabetes results from arterial disease. Alzheimer's risk is 65% higher for those with diabetes, possibly due to calcification in arteries in the brain. The risk of dementia is nearly twice as great in an elderly individual who has diabetes. Roughly one in ten with diabetes experience nerve damage. Signs of nervous dysfunction in diabetes include exercise intolerance, ventricular dysfunction of the heart, sexual impotence, and rapid heartbeat. Delayed stomach emptying is found in 1 of 2 individuals with diabetes.

The process of glycosylation is similar to the browning or toasting of food in a toaster. It is more familiar by its general name, the "Maillard" reaction.[cxc]   Injury in arteries is ultimately caused by severe rusting or oxidative stress, or oxidation, followed by widespread attack of white blood cells of these glued up arteries to try and clear the damage.[cxci] Cholesterol is just an innocent bystander. The leading cause of skin damage, oxidation, and aging, is also glycosylation, not damage from fat. One of the outward signs of high carbohydrate consumption is a significant increase of the aging process. The Maillard or "browning" reaction, leads to a process in advanced diabetes called acanthosis, a roughening and loss of elasticity of the skin. In general, the wrinkling process is due to glycosylation in the skin. The process that browns a piece of toast is similar to the one that ages and wrinkles the skin. Does this happen in hypercholesteremia. It does not. Cholesterol makes lipid membranes more elastic. Fructose from fruit and honey is actually 10 times more likely to damage arteries than glucose.[cxcii] [cxciii] Eating too much fructose accelerates aging and significantly changes the collagen in skin and bones.[cxciv] [cxcv]

The enormous oxidizing potential of fruits and grains outweighs consideration of fruit and grains for their role as valuable sources of antioxidants. From the ORAC antioxidant chart in the back of this book, one will see that vegetables outweigh grain and fruit considerably in antioxidants, almost ten to one. Grains and fruits are exponentially greater for their oxidative effects than antioxidant power. Eating fruits and grains to get antioxidants is like spilling a glass of radioactive chemicals and then trying to clean up the mess. The best antioxidant found in nature is prevention --- simply not eating large amounts of carbohydrate.

Weight loss is not a side effect of cholesterol- lowering medications. Severe muscle wasting called rhabdomyolysis and liver damage are.[cxcvi][cxcvii] Fat makes up the outer bi layer of every cell. Cholesterol and other fats increase cell fluidity, rather than their rigidity, despite common belief. Fats also form the myelin, an outer layer that surrounds and protects every nerve in the nervous system. The brain is roughly 70% fat. If fat were to oxidize faster than sugar, it would wreak havoc throughout the body, that is, in every cell of the human body and brain. The notion that butter, heavy cream, and eggs contribute to heart disease, is a common myth. These animal fats are only detrimental because antibiotics, hormones, parasites and viruses can be found in or added to them and because they are pro-inflammatory. Non animal fats high in omega three fats, omega nine or medium chain fats have no inflammation associated with them, and do not contribute to obesity or heart disease. Many lesser factors can contribute to heart disease. Omega-6 fatty acids, bacteria, viruses and alcohol. The most common forms of high triglycerides (a type of fat or "lipid" similarly formed in the liver) seen clinically are not familial hypercholesterolemia, but are found in diabetes, alcoholism, and kidney disease.[cxcviii][cxcix][cc] The major cholesterol medication class, the statins causes rhabdomyolysis, a severe and debilitating disease of the muscles. Some of these medications have been removed from market, but they still remain the drug of choice (lovastatin) for heart disease, a condition neither caused by cholesterol nor affected by it, outside a 1 in 2 million disorder. The irony is that the vast majority of cholesterol is made from carbohydrate in our diet in the liver. Fat cannot be turned into cholesterol. Clinically, vegetarians have the highest rate of triglycerides in the blood, largely because of their high carbohydrate intake, not because of their intake of fat and cholesterol. They have the highest rate along with individuals with Diabetes.

In the 1950s, Rachel Carson's "Silent Spring" was able to overturn the use of PCB pesticides. This classic work helped remove carcinogenic PCB compounds from our rivers and streams and helped launch the environmental movement. Ironically, the low carbohydrate trend in the last 15 years has gone further to wipe out the rainforest than any other diet trend. Almost 90% of our rainforests in South America have been destroyed from cattle farming.

Every year millions of hectares of tropical forest are lost due to the over consumption of meat throughout the world. Along with spiritual reasons, this may be the single largest reason against large meat consumption along with higher Cancer rates.

Between 1960 and 1990, more than 20 % of rainforests in the world disappeared. 33% percent of deforestation took place in Asia with 18% in Africa and South America. Current deforestation in the Amazon rainforest proceeds at an even greater speed today. In 11 countries, much of the remaining forests will be cleared in less than 50 years. Fifty years to wipe out the remaining forests, a truly scary thought even for the most veteran Atkins dieter. Forests are being cleared today at a rate of an acre a minute.

In Latin America, a cattle ranching is the leading cause of deforestation. Between the years 2000 and 2006, Brazil lost 150,000 square kilometers of forest, an area larger than Greece. One third of the earth's surface is dedicated to human food production.[cci] Poor farmers use fire for clearing land and every year satellite images pick up tens of thousands of fires burning across the Amazon.*[ccii] Almost 30% of the carbon dioxide released into the atmosphere yearly results from the burning of forests for local agricultural use and wood fires used for cooking. More than half of Central America's rainforests have been destroyed, in 25 years, to provide beef to North America.[cciii]

The loss of rainforests has contributed to global warming, along with fossil fuels. In 2003, 35,000 were killed by heat waves in Europe. The Himalayan Glaciers feeds seven of the world's major river systems and provides drinking water for 40% of the world's population. In the next 50 years, nearly half the world's population may face a serious water shortage if warming trends continue.[cciv] In 1998, the hottest year on record, the world lost an estimated 16% of all its coral reefs. If carbon dioxide levels continue to rise, there will be a loss of soil moisture of up to 35% in 50 years in America directly affecting our food crops and their prices.[ccv] Tsunamis are affecting much of Africa and the Middle East, and Asia. In 2004, Japan set a record for floods, with 10 typhoons. In the 1930s, protective barriers were placed on the Thames river to protect London from flooding. They closed the barriers fewer than twice from 1930 to 1980. In the 1980s closures doubled and in the 1990s, they have tripled in number.

It is our obligation to examine how a large change in diet affects our natural resources. The irony may be that choosing one way may be good for our health short-term but difficult for us and for the environment long-term. We cannot plow all our dollars into meat and dairy production without regard to preserving our delicate ecosystem and food chain. We need to find new ways to ensure that these are around for generations to come. A low carbohydrate diet may bear larger opportunity costs. We can't simply turn into lemmings, running over cliffs with each new diet. We need to carefully consider and project all the public health and ethical consequences first. An intelligent diet will endure for the long-term.

Although heart disease is a major cause of mortality, it is tied with cancer as the leading killer in America. The development of cancer is related to diet and environmental factors. In present-day agriculture, hormones used in animal farming, and pesticides used on our crops are a serious problem in terms of their effects on humans and animals. Today, even corrupt Harvard physicians with no toxicology training regularly sit on prestigious medical ethics committees preaching about the wonders of toxic chemotherapy for Cancer patients, sending these patients to their demise. They lead their hapless followers to their end.

Insulin is widely considered the single leading food based cause of cancer today, above aflatoxin, a peanut mold and even food additives. Not surprisingly, the rate of breast cancer mirrors the rate of diabetes, 1 in 10. The rate of obesity in men fairly mirrors the rate of prostate cancer, 1 in 3. Insulin is known to release estrogen from their carrier proteins, allowing them to act freely in the body. Food, primarily grains and fruit, contribute more than any other food to increased cancer risk, through their promotion of insulin, the most powerful cancer causing hormone.

Women with diabetes have a 20 per cent greater risk of developing breast cancer, according to 20 studies. [ccvi] In one combined study of American and Canadian women fewer than 50, those with the highest level of insulin like growth factor, were 7 times more likely to develop breast cancer. In over 10,000 women in Italy, older than 35, those with high blood sugar levels were three times more likely to develop breast cancer. Insulin receptors are six times higher on breast cancer cells compared to normal cells. Obese women have a 50% greater risk of cancer than lean women. Obese women, have much higher levels of insulin and free estrogen. A high level of insulin, according to Columbia University's department of oncology is the single leading risk factor for Cancer.

People with diabetes had an 82 per cent higher risk of developing pancreatic cancer (36 studies covering more than 9,000 patients). (Pollak et al. 2010) The prevalence of diabetes is high in patients with lymphoma, especially lymphoma in the head, nose and sinuses, and central nervous system. Reduced immune system function may be the cause, as high blood sugar is known to reduce the natural killer cells and neutrophils by up to 50%, one reason for high infections in diabetes. Individuals with Diabetes are roughly 30% more likely to develop colon cancer (15 studies covering 2.5 million patients). [ccvii] Another group found that for a group of men with prostate cancer, the risk was 9 times greater for those with the highest levels of IGF, insulin-like-growth factor.

Cancer cells, which are anaerobic, rely on glucose alone, unlike normal cells, which respire through fatty acid metabolism. Starving cancer cells of sugar is one of the major therapies, along with reducing exposure to insulin from diet or medication. The more carbohydrate in the diet, the more these cells are allowed to flourish. Normal oxygen rich cells use fat for ATP synthesis (fatty acids). Studies of a high carbohydrate diet with mice show that after a little over two months, over 64% of the mice died (16 of 24)on the high carbohydrate diet compared to just 1 of 20 mice with tumors on a low carbohydrate diet.

Additional studies have shown that a high glycemic index is associated with cancer of the ovaries. For years, poly cystic ovarian syndrome has been related to diabetes. Women with this disorder have chronic an-ovulation, menstrual abnormalities, and overproduction of sex hormones. The associated complications of PCOS, obesity, high triglycerides or fat in the blood, insulin resistance, and less commonly, hypertension aren't usually the reasons people seek medical care, but may be the long-term predictors of mortality and morbidity. This disorder affects 5-10% of women. It is also extremely common in women with hyperglycemia and hyperinsulinemia.[ccviii] Glucose intolerance, characterized by insulin resistance, the pre-diabetes condition, is 5-10 times higher in women with PCOS than normal.[ccix]

High glucose and insulin levels appear to contribute to high levels of androgens such as estrogen by direct effect on the ovary and the adrenals. Insulin may also lower sex hormone-binding globulin levels, allowing androgens to act freely on tissues, exerting their cancerous effects. Insulin resistance is present in virtually all PCOS patients.[ccx] High glucose and insulin are likely the same pathogenic factor for both PCOS and diabetes.

Cows that feed only on pasture do not lactate during the latter half of pregnancy. A cow becomes pregnant as a result of natural mating, milk their cows for five months, and obtain at best, around 5 liters of milk a day. In the early 1900s, as technology lowered the price of ammonia fertilizers, farmers began applying it to enable dairy farmers to use surplus crops as feed grains for cows. Today, a Modern Holstein cow with the addition of a steady diet of grains and other additives lactates for almost 305 days a year.[ccxi]

In addition to grain feeding, hormone use has also greatly increased milk and beef production as well. By drinking 300 ml of milk a day, a child's intake in Japan is approximately 10 mg of estradiol 17-B. This estradiol is the most potent estrogen and this amount is equal to 4000 times the intake of environmental hormones. High dairy consumption is a major cause of reproductive disorders in males and increased cancer rates in Japan today. [ccxii] Furthermore, pasteurization does not kill the large reservoir of parasites and viruses found in cow's milk, making milk the second leading cause of the parasite infestation, after undercooked meat or sushi. As a nomad in Mongolia once said, "If we steal too much milk from pregnant cows, they cannot give us good calves."[ccxiii]

By feeding cows estrogens, antibiotics, and growth hormones, we are seeing some of the lost fruits of our labor. Some of the diseases we suffer as a result of our actions include increased risk of Crohns disease (from antibiotic overuse with cows), prostate cancer and breast cancer. Stealing from the cows has not been without consequence.

One of the most effective treatments for Cancer today is digestive enzymes. These enzymes, such as amylase (starch digestion), proteases (protein digestion), and lipases (fat digestion), normally released from the pancreas, assist in protein breakdown in the body. Digestive enzymes appear to degrade the protective layers cancer cells create to protect themselves from the immune system. When pancreatic digestive enzymes are overtaxed, the enzymes have to come from somewhere other than the pancreas. They typically have to come from immune cells, our white blood cells. This can lead to increased allergies, decreased immunity, and even Cancer. It may also be that the more food that needs to be digested, the more energy is taken away from fighting Cancer cells, towards the digestive process. Herbivore-insectivores have a pancreas less than a third the size of humans. This is because their diet has many times the enzymes ours does because of all the high enzyme grass, vegetables, and herbs in their diet. Humans also have a pancreas much larger to accommodate their greater protein intake as Carnivores.

Vegetables such as ginger and green leafy vegetables are highest in digestive enzymes. Vegetables also are high in carotenoids such as beta-carotene, a vitamin A precursor that is found largely in green leafy vegetables. Carotenoids that help stabilize cell growth and development and are also beneficial for individuals with Cancer. The more raw vegetables in the diet, the lower the risk of Cancer. Foods with inhibition of cancer cell growth include wheat grass, garlic, brussel sprouts, scallions, leeks, broccoli, cauliflower, Savoy cabbage, onion, cabbage, kale, and spinach. Vegetable super food blends high in wheat grass and similar vegetables are considered highly beneficial for curing Cancer because of their high enzyme content. The relatively high magnesium deficiency, the most common of all vitamins and minerals, suggests most Americans are vegetable deficient.

Vegetables are many times higher in digestive enzymes, antioxidants, carotenoids, and vitamins and minerals than fruits. Cooking may destroy some of the enzymes in vegetables so many individuals with Cancer consume vegetables raw. They are higher in fiber and have almost no starch or sugar, excluding root vegetables. For this reason, any "Raw food" diet should include almost entirely vegetables, and vegetable protein, not cereal and fruit. A "raw" diet high in fruit and cereal will send insulin plummeting, likely the largest single cause of Cancer. A raw food diet, calling for lower animal protein may be helpful for someone with Cancer. But basic protein levels must be met not only for normal white blood cell production and to prevent cancer cachexia, the breakdown of body protein to support immune cell production

Small amounts of chicken, (i.e. twice a week), and meat once or twice a month, might lead to much better overall health, and lower Cancer risk than high meat protein diets. Dairy, processed meats, hot dogs, hamburgers, and the like should all be avoided in individuals with or without this disease. Most Cancer causing chemicals such as PCBs and dioxin are stored in the fat tissues of animals. Undercooked meat and dairy are also the most common sources of cancer-causing parasites, viruses, and bacteria. Many parasites and viruses are associated with Cancer. Pasteurization does not kill viruses and parasites, and on an industrial scale does a poor job of killing Mycobacteria, a hardy bacteria considered the leading cause of Crohns disease. A low carbohydrate diet that gets most of its protein from vegetarian (non-soy) choices is the most wise diet for anyone of any age, for both health and spiritual reasons. Most low carbohydrate diets send out the wrong message and people in Hollywood today are eating steak and chicken three times a day. This is not an Anti-Cancer preventive diet, or good for the environment. Obesity and heart disease are not the only killers.

A true vegetarian, consuming adequate sources of protein, fiber, vitamins and minerals, greatly promotes his or her health over a meat eater. This is the case in many eastern nations. A westernized vegetarian pursuing primarily a grain and fruit based diet stands only to increase one's risk of obesity and heart disease. Clinically, vegetarians in America have higher levels of obesity and triglycerides than non-vegetarians.

In the 1970s, Rachel Carson's book about environmental pollution, "Silent Spring" was instrumental in changing government policies in agriculture. It also led to the rise of the Environmental Protection Agency. The pesticides and other industrial chemicals she wrote of harm everything from animals as small as birds and bees to humans. Pesticides and industrial wastes still play a major role in cancer.

PCBs were invented to make plastics more pliable, and had been banned since the 1970s, two decades after Rachel Carson's book on the subject. PCBs are members of a family of 219 toxic chemicals that can damage the immune system and the hormones of humans and other animals. They lead to infertility, and cancer, disrupting endocrine systems, and known to promote hermaphroditic fish and polar bears. A study of fulmar carcasses washed ashore on North Sea coastlines found that 95% had plastic in their stomachs, an average of 44 pieces per bird. These plastics attract PCBs and toxic chemicals in birds, and puffins swallowing plastic have concentrated poisons in their fat tissues as high as 1 million times their concentration in seawater.[ccxiv] PCBs acts like sponges for DDT, and other fat-soluble toxins. When they enter the human food chain, their concentration multiplies even further. However, PCB use still remains widespread. DDT, and Dieldren are forty times more toxic than PCBs.[ccxv]

The scientists today are like the false prophets and magicians, in Pharaoh's palace. They are turning the Nile red, with food colorings and genetic engineered produce.

Modern medicine has become stagnant as the Dead Sea, a selfish sea, corrupt and putting profits first. Autism is affecting 1 in 200, compared to 1 in 20,000 twenty years ago. Millions of birds are falling out of the air due to unknown causes, oil fills the waters, and tsunamis are striking at will. The male sperm, due to malnutrition, chemicals and possibly rising age of procreation, have caused autism to skyrocket. This may be the second largest epidemic after diabetes.

In 1976, an accident at a Hoffman-LaRoche pesticide factory in Seveso, Italy, spewed dioxin into the surrounding community. A cloud of chemicals was released into the air and eventually contaminated an area of 15 square kilometers with a population of 37,000 people. They have suffered a variety of serious long-term effects including increased incidence of cancer, including cancers of the stomach and rectum, leukemia (cancer of the blood-forming cells) and lymphomas. One contamination case in the U.S. a few years ago resulted from the use of clay as a binder in chicken feed. In 1998, Sterling Chemical expelled a cloud of benzene that hospitalized hundreds, following a leak of ammonia in 1994 that injured almost 10,000 In 1999, Belgian health authorities examined poultry, eggs, beef, pork, milk, and found traces of Dioxin and other highly cancerous poly-chlorinated biphenyl substances known as PCBs. The Dutch Ministry of Health notified the Belgians that they had measured dioxin in two chickens at 958 and 775 parts per trillion toxic equivalents. In Belgium, the allowable limit for dioxin in chicken is 5 part per trillion toxic equivalents. In the U.S. the limit is one part per trillion. The problem was traced to 8 liters of oil containing PCBs contaminated with 50 to 80 milligrams of dioxin. Toxic oil was taken from an electrical transformer and dumped illegally into a public recycling container used to collect used cooking oil. The contaminated oil ended up in an 88-ton (80 metric tons) batch of fat produced by Verkest, a company located near Ghent, Belgium. The fat was sold to 12 manufacturers of animal feed, who then produced 1760 tons (1600 metric tons) of contaminated

animal feed. Starting in January, 1999, the feed was sold
mainly in Belgium but also in France and the Netherlands.
A plant in Chocolate Bayou, Texas that makes acrylonitrile
was 2002's biggest releaser of carcinogens in the United
States.[ccxvi] In 2005, BP, British Petrol, released a geyser of
liquid hydrocarbons into the air, killing 15 people. In July,
2005, a hydrogen pipe exploded, followed by a hydrogen
sulfide leak a month later, shutting much of BP down. A
plastics plant exploded days later. They were the named
2006's biggest polluter.

Chemotherapy, the current medical treatment for Cancer,
is one of the most lethal in conventional medicine, ranking
highest along with blood pressure medications and
NSAIDS. It is also one of the least effective, with
approximately a 2% success rate. Most successful cures
for Cancer are botanical and other naturopathic remedies.
Today, toxicity from medical drugs is the third leading
cause of death in the country. Drug side effects are the
fourth leading cause of death in the world. In 1994,
2,216,000 hospitalized patients had serious adverse drug
reactions and 106,000 died from them.[ccxvii] Medications
annually kill more than 100,000 Americans. In 2002,
16,176 adverse drug reaction reports were received, of
which 67% were serious.[ccxviii] Drug-related morbidity and
mortality have been estimated to cost more than $136
billion a year in United States. These estimates are higher
than the total cost of cardiovascular or diabetes care in the
United States. [ccxix] In a survey of over 28,000 patients,
advanced drug reactions were considered to be the cause of
3.4 percent of hospital admissions. Of these, 187 were
reviewed as severe. The four drugs most frequently
responsible for adverse drug reactions are diuretics, calcium
channel blockers, non-steroidal anti-inflammatory drugs,
and digoxin.[ccxx] The major cholesterol medication class, the
statins causes rhabdomyolysis, a severe and debilitating
disease of the muscles. Some of the medications in this
class have been removed from market, but they still remain
the drug of choice (lovastatin) for heart disease, a condition

neither caused by cholesterol nor affected by it, outside a 1 in 2 million disorder.

In medical school, they were taking a patient who had a t-cell lymphoma in a Harvard hospital, and the medical student is told she is getting comfort care. They are giving her comfort care, which means methotrexate (ie. Mustard gas). Her disease is "Genetic", the young resident will say to the student. (something doctors say when they don't have an answer. There is no investigation for viruses, parasites, and chemicals that may play a role in this Cancer. The medical student checks on the computer on "pubmed" database and finds 16,000 entries for two parasites suspected in t-cell lymphoma. This is intuition, as Steve Jobs would say. The student didn't consciously know these parasites caused t-cell lymphoma. He knows only that parasites were a theory in some cancers. But medicine today follows a strict protocol for Cancer, dropping a nuclear bomb, called chemotherapy. Medicine does not reward Physicians for creativity, ingenuity, or novel thinking. It is difficult to be a thinking, common sense, intuitive person in medicine, because the goal is not helping the patient find out what is causing their disease. It is following a protocol, and putting a band-aid on the patient. People rate modern medicine as the most respected profession in one large magazine poll. If they were on the inside, they would see, that medicine is as prone to corruption as banks and law firms.

The average Harvard medical student will see the drug side effects in their medical school books, but they will learn as an instinct eventually not to see them. One or two with a conscience, a light burning inside, might want to speak up in class, but are afraid to rock the boat. They sense a small light bulb go on, when they see all the side effects are many times worse, than the condition. But something gets in the way, the prestige perhaps, the money. Ethics are not taught at Harvard medical school.

In 2003, drug makers removed a decongestant phenylpropanolamine from popular cold medicines due to the risk of stroke and brain hemorrhaging in infants. At least 1,500 children under age 2 required emergency room care in 2004 and 2005 after taking non-prescription cough and cold medicines. Another review conducted for the FDA documented 54 deaths involving decongestants and 69 involving antihistamines from 1969 to 2006. Among the deaths, most occurred in children younger than two. In October 2007, more than 14 popular infant cold and flu formulas were removed from the market altogether. Medications today turn up in the tissue of the fish we eat, signs that they have entered our water supplies and affect our public health even when we do not take medications. Today, Naturopathic Schools of Medicines have begun to develop in many states in response to the revealed toxicity of most pharmaceuticals.

5 Ten Steps to Greatness

Across the world, nearly 1 billion people find themselves in desperate need of food. Five million children under the age of five die every year as a result of going hungry. We have the ability to feed everyone. The world produces 20% more food than is even consumed.

Rainforest land yields the landowner $60 per acre for cattle and $400 per acre for timber. If the renewable and sustainable resources were harvested instead, the land would yield the landowner $2,400 per acre. The 2000-2001 World Resources Report by the UN suggests that governments worldwide spend $700 billion dollars a year supporting and subsidizing environmentally nonrenewable, unethical and unwise practices.[ccxxi] Poultry and fish are far less energy intensive to raise than cows. Poultry requires less land and is four times more able to convert feed into food. Legumes require one-tenth the land required to rear animals. Americans currently consume almost a quarter of the world's beef and release one third of the world's greenhouse gasses.

Meat production also currently requires 2500 gallons of water. More than one third of North America is taken up with grazing (grass feeding). The water that goes into a 1000-pound steer would float a navy Destroyer. The requirements in cattle production have dried up many of the underground wells in dry regions of America, Australia, and other countries.[ccxxii]

Centuries ago rainforests covered more than 15% of the earth. They now cover less than 8% of the planet. Careless governments allow logging companies to clear this land by means of chainsaws, bulldozers and fires. They sell the land to farming operations.[ccxxiii] Rain forests assure the preservation of water, healthy soil, plants and animal life. These forests also help to regulate global temperature and rainfall. Many plants are valuable for therapeutic purposes and yet undiscovered ones disappear every year.

When rainforests disappear, so do a source of their most valuable foods. These are necessary to their survival. Some vegetables from the rainforests also have very high amounts of protein. These include: mongongo nuts (28.8% protein), tsin beans (31.6%), marula nuts (30.9%), and baobab nuts (34.1%). [ccxxiv] Much of the rainforests we lose today is due to cattle farming. Before the American Southwest was settled, it was fertile grassland. After humans moved westward and the cattle population of a half million in the Southwest grew by six times, the result was a region that is still scorched with unprecedented drought, like today's Sahara.

The rainforests, which once covered all of Borneo, have all but disappeared. These forests have been cleared in recent years for logging and agriculture. Today, it has accelerated to meet the booming demand for palm oil. Palm oil is found in one in every 10 products on supermarket shelves. Ironically, the drive for bio-fuel is partly to blame as palm oil is one of the popular alternative fuels to replace petroleum. [ccxxv] Over fishing, pollution, and loss of marine biodiversity may cause fish to be depleted by 2050. [ccxxvi]

Many farms raise free- range grass fed animals. This includes proper living conditions for animals and humane slaughtering. A 1988 report by the Department of Agriculture listed 140,471 dogs, 42,271 cats, 51,641 primates, 431,457 guinea pigs, 331,945 hamsters, 459,254 rabbits, and 178,249 "wild animals", a total of 1,635,288 used in experimentation. Over 90,000 were estimated to experience unrelieved pain. In Japan, a survey in 1988 produced a total animal estimate of an excess of 8,000,000 animals were used for experimentation. [ccxxvii] Many health students witness abuses in animal rights, human drug testing, and use of harmful medications in hospitals without protest. We need to change the culture that accepts these practices. We need more inspections of our universities to uphold the twenty-year old Animal Welfare Act. We need to restrict the health care system's use of pharmaceuticals to critical and emergency care where alternatives may not exist. A legal challenge issued against Monsanto, a multinational agriculture company, revealed that animals fed its genetically modified corn suffered liver and kidney damage after three months. When buying produce we can stick to organic (not sprayed with pesticides), non-genetically engineered vegetables from smaller local markets. Pesticides harm us not only physically but are also reducing many of our most important crops by reducing the pollinating birds, and bees, vital to their continuation. Genetically engineered corn has also been shown to reduce butterfly and insect populations.

The current practice of bringing grains to countries potentially affected by food shortage is a short-term solution. A wiser and healthful policy would be working the land to yield vegetables and legumes that are indigenous to the land of the particular country, suitable for the particular conditions of that country. . Nobody in India in the 1960s thought many areas of the country would ever be fertile. Norman Borlaug, an American agronomist helped turn many barren fields into green ones. Today a team of business students, working in rural India is running small power plants on rice husks.[ccxxviii]

Written off for centuries as useless, Embrapa, Brazil's agricultural and livestock agency, has transformed 1000 miles of dry savannah in central Brazil into a major agricultural belt. He discovered that enriching the soils with a mixture of phosphorous and lime, made them fertile again. In Israel, a new category of fruit called "environmentally friendly fruit" has been developed that uses minimal chemicals to prevent local ecosystems from being disrupted.[ccxxix] Advances in Israel's water irrigation, now enables crops to be grown with less than half the water in the past. Every seven years, the entire land is set aside to lay fallow for one year. This ensures that the land remains fertile for times to come, the needy are allowed take what they wish, and leftovers are provided to the animals.

We've learned recently how overuse of ethanol and palm oil, causes enormous loss of rainforest. Today, solar energy is providing energy without any loss of natural resources. It is also proving itself profitable in Japan and other countries after initial subsidization. In Japan, vision and philosophy and business sense are not mutually exclusive. On some nights in Denmark, the winter winds meet all the needs for energy along the coast. By 2008, one quarter of the country's electricity will come from windmills. Wind power has become Denmark's largest export.[ccxxx]

Today, when US and People magazine bombard us with idols for success and happiness, we are a generation with less self-esteem than ever. However, clearly the fall of many of Hollywood's finest today shows us that wealth, and fame are not enough to make a person happy. The most effective program for addiction today has become Alcoholics Anonymous. This has nothing to do with alchohol but because one needs to have an element of spirituality in a program to address the root cause of addiction. This means more than making note of the mind-body connection, finding the mind-soul connection. According to the Lubavitcher Rebbe, good health is only found through the pursuit of spiritual health. A commitment to healing through abiding by commandments in Torah offers an infinitely more powerful approach than manmade solutions in science and psychology. Torah provides not just lessons for life, but the very blueprint for emotional and physical health. Many say we don't need G-d in these advanced technological times. Yet our inventions have brought us no closer to relief from hunger, poverty, disease, war, or crime. We need G-d more than ever. Sometimes it is only in the greatest darkness of night that someone finally can see the stars.

Nations have always turned to the East for answers. Some turn to India, others Tibet, some meditate on mountaintops or pray at the Western Wall in Jerusalem. Some like the Dalai Lama, others Deepak Chopra or comparable Jewish healers. There was recently a Jewish woman who was stricken with a serious illness who travelled to the far East, to ask a renowned Indian healer for answers. The healer told her, "You Jewish people are always sitting on your own great rivers of healing and yet always seem to believe the answers are found in someone else's backyard. Go to the Western wall, and pray there. "When will you be healed?," she said. When the Jewish people get their act together and return to G-d, then the world will find its healing." [ccxxxi] Only G-d heals and saves us. "Our task is to illuminate the shadows. Each illumination small or large changes the world. " [ccxxxii]

The ten step program for healing has as its source, the Jewish spiritual and ethical teachings of the mussar movement, in 19th century Eastern Europe. The Hebrew word Mussar means instruction, discipline, or conduct. This movement made significant contribution to Jewish ethics in a time when rational "enlightenment", "science", and "innovation" were threatening to pull people away from ethics and Torah. Many call Rabbi Salanter, the father of "Psychology" and the first to develop the concept of the "Subconscious", before this idea was popularized by Sigmund Freud. These ideas were passed on to the first modern Psychologists such as Carl Jung. Although Jung was not Jewish, he transmitted these ideas to the founders of the original Steps program to help combat alcoholism. He feared that telling others G-d and spirituality was the key to addiction wouldn't go over well and would not sell. But today this method is the most successful program in the world for healing addiction.

The Ten Steps:

Step #1: We admit that we are powerless and that only a Power greater than ourselves can restore us to health physically and emotionally.

Step #2: Make a moral inventory and admit our mistakes to G-d.

Step #3: Admit to G-d and to ourselves the exact nature of our wrongs and how we would like to commit to improving ourselves. And.that we are entirely ready to have G-d remove and assist us with these improvements of character.

Step #4: Humbly ask Him to remove and forgive us our shortcomings.

Step #5: Make a list of all persons we have harmed, and make amends to them all with an apology.

Step #6: Make direct amends to such people wherever possible, except when to do so would injure them or others.

Step #7: Express gratitude for the blessings in our life, health, children, wealth, etc.

Step #8: Through prayer and meditation, seek to improve your connection to G-d

Step #10: Having had a spiritual uplifting as the result of these steps, carry this message to others with the same addiction or problem as ourselves, and implement these steps into daily life and personal prayer. .

Simply curing one's overeating or any form of addiction is not a simple process. The evil inclination that whispers to a person--- you can start tomorrow--- is not so easily defeated. If this were as simple as a physical addiction, one could simply take away the offender for three days (sugar or alcohol) and allow the addiction three days to dry out. Following the side effects of withdrawal, a clear-thinking person would not want to return to the addiction. So why doesn't it work this way? [ccxxxiii]Torah says that the real addict is trying to essentially fill a spiritual void or vacuum. The real problem today isn't junk food. It is a junk lifestyle devoid of spiritual purpose, selfless kindness, and meaning. Alcohol or food is what is used to drown out a larger unperceived anxiety of being no longer connected to a higher spiritual source. The only means to cure the addiction is therefore not the drug but by reconnecting to the spiritual source, Torah and its commandments. And this is why statistics for heart disease and addiction are much lower when the individual connects through spiritual places, such as prayer or support groups. The true anorexia today is therefore a spiritual anorexia. The more course and crass the world has become, the more we crave structure and spiritual guidance. As the outside world has become corrupt and dishonest, we come to seek greater light and wisdom. Once we tap into this spiritual wisdom, our hunger diminishes, and our real craving is appeased. Teens sitting in diners across America are coming back to their faith, when they realize cheeseburgers and shakes are not real soul food. The more we grow spiritually, the more your self-esteem will grow and one's health blossoms.

What happened when we took the study of ethics out of the schools in the 1960s? Crime soared. Drug use, teenage pregnancy, smoking, and alcohol use rose dramatically.[ccxxxiv] People in this country are always saying, " It's not fair. Why am I sick? Why am I struggling with such trials and tribulations? It isn't fair." There is actually no word in the Hebrew language for "fair," which is subjective. There is right, and there is wrong. All the isms today are dead. The one ism that has prevailed is the Torah. It is the most powerful and unknown river for healing.[ccxxxv] Today, our education makes ethics an afterthought. And every business, including the banks, law firms, and medical schools are affected. They don't teach ethics at Harvard Medical School. Whether a fence is metal or wood, it needs to be painted. A metal fence that isn't painted rusts. And a wood fence begins to rot. Judaism compares a fence to our soul. And just as with our soul, we need to do everything we can to protect it and guard it to achieve greatness.[ccxxxvi]

An American soldier turned lawyer once interviewed a
Jewish law school graduate for a prestigious job in a top
law firm. The lawyer was impressed because it said on the
graduate's resume that he had studied the Jewish Talmud.
The hiring lawyer told him that there was only one thing he
feared in life, an Israeli soldier. "Why is that?" asked the
young Jewish law graduate? "Because an Israeli soldiers, he
said, spend years in battle figuring out who they are, and
years figuring out their enemy." The young graduate was
hired. Before you can know yourself, you have to know
your strengths and weaknesses. And before you can
succeed, you must know your enemy even better. A
successful battle plan for health takes preparation as much
spiritual as physical. When the wise King Solomon was
asked what he most wanted in life, he did not ask for fame,
for wealth, honor, or might. He asked for a "knowing
heart." A knowing heart means understanding how to
appreciate wisdom and apply it. The key to happiness in
life involves knowing who you are, and knowing your
enemy. In the old days, the great students of the Jewish
ethics, were immersed in the study of ethics all day long.
The wife of Rabbi Kanievsky, one of the great spiritual
leaders of the century once asked him to make a cup of
coffee. He responded, "First tell me what coffee is, and
then tell me how to make it." She said to him, "You are
the master of Jewish law, and you don't know how to make
coffee?." He answered," It is because I have spent my life
studying the entire work of the Talmud, that I don't know
how to make a cup of coffee. If I knew how to make
coffee, I would not know the entire Talmud." Rabbi
Povarsky, a wise Torah sage, once asked his grandchild, to
show him to his kitchen. His wife had just passed away,
and his grandchild asked, "You don't know where the
kitchen is?" The Rabbi replied, "My mother said to me, if
you want to become a scholar, don't ever go into the
kitchen. I listened to her." The purpose and mission of life
is not our success. It is how we reach our potential.[ccxxxvii]

This means understanding our strengths and our
weaknesses and creating a successful battleplan to reach

our potential. Rather than focus on your shortcomings, focus on your strengths. Make one small resolution than many big ones. Start you're your physical health. Without one's physical health, there can be no spiritual health. The Chassidic saying is "A small hole in the body creates a larger hole in the soul.". For example you wouldn't feed your child a donut and coffee for breakfast. Try a week where you simply start your child's day with a healthy breakfast for a change and first work on improving your family's physical health before starting your spiritual growth. Spend more time helping an elderly parent or relative, and you will see how this translates into your own health. The word spiritual in Hebrew comes from the word ruach or "wind", something that isn't seen. Why something not seen? Because it is often the small act of kindness that make a large impact. Even the dark side of the moon pulls the tides. The Lubavitcher Rebbe says, there are two ways to cure an illness. One is to heal the particular organ or faculty that is weak or sick. The other is to strengthen the healthy organs and faculties so that they may overcome and heal the sick organ or faculty.[ccxxxviii] The parallel approach spiritually, he says, is teshuvah (return or personal accounting) and small good deeds.

Let the sunshine in. The word depression and lazy share the same root in the Hebrew language. The lowest spiritual level a person can reach is depression. Rather than letting life get us down, we need to simply turn our bitterness into movement. The Hebrew word for healthy "bari" comes from the same root as the word "asbara", which means to be creative. When we are healthy, we can produce and be creative. To serve our mission here, we need to have energy and passion. As the Chassidic saying goes, "Think good and it will be good." If we really want to make a lasting change in the world, we have to first change ourselves. As we change ourselves, we change our family. Our family can change our city. And this is how we change the world.

A study was recently done on people who said they planned to stop drinking. Those that started that day were ten times more likely a year later to have quit than those who put it off until the next day or beyond. [ccxxxix] In Judaism, there is no such thing as putting off the now. We must nurture in ourselves and others the courage to live and act in the now. If everyone said "I love you" to their wife today, started the job they really want to live today, and began their diet today, the world would be a better place. Rabbi Akiva, at the age of 40 went from a humble peasant to study in yeshiva and become the greatest Torah scholar the world ever knew. As Rabbi Akiva shows, it's never too late. What was it that made him return to school at the age of 40? He realized that if the very nature of a stone could be changed slowly with the passing of water over it, then man's heart could also undergo dramatic change and inner renewal, through small daily effort. As one slow passing of the river over the stone, one thought turns into action, the action becomes our habit, and our habit becomes our character. The distance to good health may seem like a large river to cross. But it's really as easy as turning one's direction from east to west, often one simple change of perspective. We are standing on the river.

A Diet for a Little Planet

The Answer: The Quick Users Guide

Grain, Fruit, Sugar →

Carbohydrate →

Glucose (sugar) →

Glycerol Phosphate (sugar derivative) →

Triglyceride (Fat)
Fat   (Fatty Acids plus Glycerol) X ---(CANNOT) →
Triglyceride (Fat)

(Exact pathway)

Grains or fruit →Carbohydrate (sugar or starch) →
Glucose (sugar) → acetyl Coa→ fatty acids
(With fatty acid synthase)

Grains or fruit →Carbohydrate (sugar or starch) →
Glucose (sugar) → glycerol 3 phosphate* (sugar
derivative) + fatty acids = adipose triglyceride or fat
(*Rate-limiting reagent)

Triglyceride (fat) → fatty acids + glycerol(recycled to
liver) ≠ adipose triglyceride or fat

But…..

Triglyceride (fat) → Glycerol → ≠ Triglyceride
(Fat)

Insulin: Lock and Key System of Body

Insulin → Locks in Body Fat and Water (H20)
(hormone stimulated by glucose)

Glucagon ← Releases Fat, H20 (stimulated by protein)

The Ten Step Program

Step #1: We admit that we are powerless and that only a Power greater than ourselves can restore us to health physically and emotionally.

Step #2: Make a moral inventory and admit our mistakes to G-d.

Step #3: Admit to G-d and to ourselves the exact nature of our wrongs and how we would like to commit to improving ourselves. And.that we are entirely ready to have G-d remove and assist us with these improvements of character.

Step #4: Humbly ask Him to remove and forgive us our shortcomings.

Step #5: Make a list of all persons we have harmed, and make amends to them all with an apology.

Step #6: Make direct amends to such people wherever possible, except when to do so would injure them or others.

Step #7: Express gratitude for the blessings in our life, health, children, wealth, etc.

Step #8: Through prayer and meditation, seek to improve your connection to G-d

Step #10: Having had a spiritual uplifting as the result of these steps, carry this message to others with the same addiction or problem as ourselves, and implement these steps into daily life and personal prayer. .

The Top Ten Ten Pound Weight Loss Answers

Cereal   Up to 40 grams per serving
Bread (whole grain or processed) and Rolls, bagels, muffins, etc. Up to 40 grams per serving
Orange juice (Grape juice, Apple juice, etc.) Up to 80 grams in one glass
Crackers   Up to 40 grams per serving
Donuts   Up to 60 grams per donut
Cookies   Up to 40 grams per serving
Cake   Up to 60 grams per serving
Pizza   Up to 60 grams per serving
Carbonated soft drinks   Up to 60 grams per can
Chocolate Milk   Up to 40 grams per glass

Factored in are total combined yearly consumption patterns of Americans and total carbohydrate content of food and drinks.

Top 5 Healthy Foods

Small Fish
Hangar Steak (Lean red meat)
Beets
Cabbage (Green leafy vegetables)
Stomach
Cow's Womb
(According to Talmud, Tractate Brochas, foods which heal
and can restore a sick person to good health)

Least 5 Healthy Foods

Fatty Meat
Eggs
Dairy
Most Nuts
Poultry

(According to Talmud, Tractate Brochas foods which make
one ill, and make one who is sick, more ill)

In Moderation

Grain   One serving a day
Fruit   In limitation (According to Maimonides)
i.e. One serving a day
Legumes—Lentils, Black beans, Kidney beans, etc.
Seeds—pumpkin, sesame
Some nuts-- Almonds, walnuts

Carbohydrate and Fiber Contents in Food

(For actual starch content subtract fiber from carbohydrate)

GRAIN

Starch (Grams),Fiber Content (Grams)

Pancake Betty Crocker 3 pancakes	39, 1
Shredded wheat Arrowhead	38, 2
Rice, white, Uncle Ben's Long grain ¼ cup	38,0
Barley, pearled cup Arrowhead Mills	32,1
Rice, brown Arrowhead Long grain	32, 1
Cookies 4 Chips Ahoy Cookies Nabisco	28, 0
F-Factor Cereal with Apples,Raspberries	**27,18**
Oatmeal Half cup Quaker Oats	27, 4
Bran muffin piece Hodgson Mill	27, 3
Brownie piece Entenmann's	25, 1
Animal cookie 16 pieces Austin Zoo	25, 0
Fiber One Cereal third cup	**24, 13**
Cheerios cup	22, 3
White Bread Pepperidge Farm 1 slice	16, 0
Whole wheat bread 9 grain "	15,3
Puffed kashi 1 cup	15, 1
Rye bread whole kernel 1 slice	16, 3

DAIRY

98% fat free ice cream Breyers chocolate	40, 4
Frozen Yogurt Chocolate Stonyfield	38, 1
Ice cream Breyers	34, 2
Dove dark chocolate bar	20, 2
Hershey bar with almonds	20, 1
Milk, 2% Organic Valley 16 oz	24, 0
Coconut cream yogurt (plain-nondairy)	**16**
Yogurt, plain Dannon low-fat	14, 0

ROOT VEGETABLES

Baked potato 1 baked 4 ¾ X 2 1/3	51, 4.8
French fries McDonalds, medium size	46, 5
Potato chips Lays original baked 1 oz.	23,2
Hash browns 3 oz. Cascadian Farm	17, 2
Mashed potato 1/3 cup mix	17,1
Potato chips Lays original	15,1
Carrots 3 carrots, chopped 7 inch	24, 6
Corn 2.3 half cup kernels gold or white	20.6,2.3

BEVERAGES

Grape juice, Organic	80, 0
Grapefruit Knudson Ruby Red	70,0
Chocolate milk (16 oz.)	64,0
Orange juice Ocean Spray	62,0
Coca cola (16 oz.)	52, 0
Snapple Ice Tea Snapple Lemon Regular	50, 0
PowerAde	32,0
Honest Tea Black Forest Berry	**16,0**
Zico Coconut water	**13,0**
Almond Milk Unsweetened choc or van	**3,0**
SoDelicious Coconut Milk, 1 cup	**1,0**

FRUIT

Mango 1 medium Dole	34,2
Date Dole 1.4 oz dried	33,3
Raisins quarter cup Dole	31,2
Banana 1 medium Dole	29,4
Prunes quarter cup Dole	26,2
Pear 1 medium Dole	25,4
Grapes 1 ½ cups Dole	24,1
Apple 1 5.4 oz. Dole Apple	22,5
Orange 1 Dole orange	21,7
Blueberries *	18
Peach 1 medium	15
Fig 1 large fig	12.3,2.1
Strawberries	**10**
Raspberries 1 cup	**7**
Lemon 1 lemon squeezed in water	**4**

Baby Food Nutrition

Vegetable Turkey Dinner 4 oz jar   10 grams carb
(61.1% carb)

Baby Food Squash 4 oz jar   7 grams carb
(87.5% carb)

Apples and Cherries 4 oz jar   4 grams carb
(94.1% carb)

Total meal Carbohydrate   21 grams carb
(79.7% carb)

Comparison Meals

Carbohydrate Total and Blood Sugar Levels

Breakfast

BETTER CHOICE

All Bran with raspberries and Almond milk
or 1 slice bread
Egg white Omelette
Israeli salad--- tomato pepper onion

Total carbohydrate   24

 Blood sugar rise over three meals:
72 micrograms/dl over baseline   (60-90 is normal baseline
blood sugar)
(average rise is 3micrograms per deciliter per gram of
carbohydrate but can be more depending on individual
metabolism)

POOR CHOICE	Carb Grams
Orange juice	62
Cereal—Oatmeal 3 grain maple raisin 1 pack	60
Milk 16 oz	24
Orange juice 16 oz	62
Multigrain bagel	57
Banana	29

Total carbohydrate

Blood sugar rise over three meals:
882 microgram/dl added to baseline (60-90 normal)

Lunch

BETTER CHOICE

Salmon	0-5
Spinach salad	0-5
Walnuts	10
Snapple Red Tea	15

Total carbohydrate	35

Blood sugar rise over three meals:
105 micrograms/dl rise over baseline (60-90 normal)

POOR CHOICE

Tuna Sandwich with two slices	30
bread whole wheat 9- grain Pepperidge Farm	
Frozen yogurt	38
Grape juice 1 glass	80

Total carbohydrate	148

Blood sugar rise over three meals:
448 micrograms over baseline (60-90 normal)

Dinner

BETTER CHOICE

Fish	0-5
Lettuce salad with olives roasted red peppers	0-5
Raspberries and walnuts	5-10
Club soda	0

Total carbohydrate	30

Blood sugar rise over three meals:
90 mg/dl   rise over baseline (60-90 normal)

POOR CHOICE

Pasta with chicken 4 oz.	85.2
2 rolls	30
Grapefruit juice	70

Total carbohydrate	185

Blood sugar rise over three meals:
555 micrograms/dl rise over baseline (60-90 normal)

Eat That Not This!?
Grams Carbohydrate

Grape juice	80
4 dove chocolate bars	80
1 packet Oatmeal	60
3 Hershey Chocolate bars with almonds	60
Mango	34
Ice cream	34
Baked potato	51
Coca cola	51
3 Carrots	24
1 Entenmann's brownie	25
Raisin Bran Cereal 1 cup	45
Crispy Cream Donut, blueberry	43
Captain Crunch Cereal 1 and half cup	44

Low Carbohydrate Sources of Vitamin C

	Milligrams Vit C
Pepper, half cup	174.8
Broccoli, half cup	123.4
Brussels sprouts,1 cup	96
Strawberry, 1 cup	81.6
Pomegranate, 100 g	62
Lemons, juice two lemons	56
Cisco fish roe/caviar (eggs)	49.6 mg/100
Grapefruit, half	46.9
Mountain sorrel (leaves and stem)	41.57/100g
Beluga caviar	6mg/100g
Kelp (seaweed)	28.36 mg/g
Blueberry	26.2/100g

* A cup of white tea has 50 times more antioxidants than a bowl of blueberries.

Antioxidants

Vegetables: (ORAC score per 100 grams)

Kale – 11770
Spinach – 11260
Brussels sprout – 1980
Alfalfa sprouts – 1930
Broccoli Flowers – 1890
Beets – 1840
Red bell pepper – 1710
Onion – 1450
Corn – 1400
Eggplant -- 1390   (legumes not included)

Fruits:

Wolfberry, Ningxia, dried   30,300
Wolfberry, Chinese   20,200
Acai   18,400
Raspberry, Black   16,400
Pomegranate   10,500
Prunes – 5570
Raisins -- 2830
Blueberries -- 2400
Blackberries -- 2036
Strawberries -- 1540
Raspberries -- 1220
Plums -- 949
Oranges -- 750
Red grapes -- 739
Cherries -- 670
Kiwi fruit -- 602
Grapefruit, pink – 483

Top Antioxidant Foods, Discovery of the Ultimate Super
food by Gary Young ND, Ronald Lawrence MD, PhD,
Marc Schreuder; Essential Science Publishing; © July 2005.
P. 48 And Tufts University

Recommended Foods

Vegetables:
Broccoli
Asparagus
Cauliflower
Squash
Beets
Brussels sprouts
Celery
Garlic
Eggplant
Spinach
Artichoke
Small Cucumbers
Pickle
Lettuce
Mushrooms
Peppers
Tomatoes
Leafy greens—kale, collard, broccoli, mustard
Raw leafy greens--- endive, escarole, radicchio, argali, frisse
Sprouts—broccoli, sunflower, radish
Sea vegetables—kelp, dulse, nori, Kombu, hijiki
Wheat or barley grass juice (fresh pressed or capsules)

Beans and legumes:
Lentils
Miso broth
Black beans
Chickpeas (hummus, falafel)
Black eyed peas
White beans
Red kidney beans
Great Northern Beans
Pinto beans

Nuts and seeds:
Walnuts
Almonds
Sunflower
Pumpkin
Flax

Condiments:
Salsa
Guacamole
Sea salt
Apple cider vinegar
Mustard
Mayonnaise
Soy sauce
Pickled ginger
Wasabi
Chermoula
Ginger paste
Green Masala
Harissa
Za'Atar
Chickpea Eggplant Dip
Beet Ginger Chutney
Piri Piri
Barbeque Sauce
Satay
Thyme Roasted Garlic
Tomato Sauce
White Bean Puree
Dairy free Yogurt Dip

Fruit:
Lemon
Lime
Raspberries
Acai berries
Grapefruit
Apple
Pomegranate

Fish: (small fish preferred)
Salmon
Scrod
Haddock
Pompano
Trout
Herring
Whitefish
Cod
Grouper
Mahi Mahi
Wahoo
Mackerel
Sole
St. Peters
St. Denis

Poultry (hormone free, free range): once to twice weekly
Chicken
Turkey
Cornish hen

Meat (leanest, organic grass fed hormone, antibiotic free) once weekly
Lean Beef-- (i.e. hangar steak)
Lamb
Venison
Buffalo

Fats and oils: (organic recommended)
Avocado or Apricot kernel (cooking)
Coconut extra virgin (cooking and therapeutic)
Extra virgin olive oil (not cooking)
Expeller pressed sesame oil
Canola (cooking)
Fish (therapeutic)

Beverages:
Herbal tea organic
Raw wheatgrass juice
Organic decaf coffee
Natural sparkling water, no carbonation added (Perrier)
Unsweetened almond milk

Sweeteners:
Unheated Raw Honey – not for infants
Stevia
Coconut syrup
Molasses

Fiber supplement:
Psyllium (0 carb)
Pectin (0 carb)
Fiber One Cereal (10 g carb/bowl)-- has aspartame
F-Factor Cereal

Vitamin C Supplement:
Lemons (by the bag)

Recommended Meal Plans

For the environment: 10-30 grams a day
- A high red meat and dairy diet destroys rainforests, and the birds and bees vital to our food supplies. It affects our pollination of crops, and pollutes vital water supplies.
- Most pesticides and dioxins are stored in animal fat. Because of all the hormones found in animals reared for market, and in the dairy supply, it is recommended that the majority of protein in the diet come from vegetables and fish.
-. A diet high in vegetable protein (i.e. tofu, legumes), fish, and moderate organic free range poultry, is the most ideal human diet. It is high in fiber, vitamins and minerals, antioxidants, protein and omega three fats. A diet high in grain and fruit is the way humans store fat and water, a way of eating not compatible with a regular diet but for periods of migration, starvation and water shortage. Humans are Carnivores. We were not made to eat cereal and fruit, like all Carnivores were not.
--- Many are returning to a vegetarian diet. Whereas the typical Western vegetarian eats pasta, potatoes, and bread, Eastern and Middle Eastern vegetarians are eating vegetables, tofu, seaweed, seeds, nuts, legumes. These foods are much higher in digestive enzymes, and beta carotene, both found to lower cancer risk. Vegetarians need to supplement with methionine. Vegans require supplementation in their diet with B-12, from brewer's yeast, or a supplement. Sea vegetables do not contain B-12, a popular misconception.

For Developing nations: 10-30 grams a day
Diabetes affects the poor and developing nations of the world even more than affluent nation. When we export grain crops rather we are exporting diabetes and obesity. Protein and vegetable crops cost more than grain crops. Getting nations to shift production of cereal grain to legumes and vegetables will help developing nations avoid Diabetes. Protein malnutrition remains in many of the poor nations despite cereal grain supplementation.

For Diabetes: 10-30 grams
-1 in 4 has high blood sugar. 1 in 11 has prediabetes. And 1 in 16 has diabetes. Diabetes is epidemic and pandemic. Each gram raises blood sugar 3 points. An average American consumes 150 grams a day, 15 times the amount required. The body is not made out of sugar but is made of protein, fat, and water. Humans are carnivores. Protein provides all the blood sugar needs for all carnivores, meaning all human beings. Ten grams is more than sufficient as a basic requirement. The body stores plenty of carbohydrate in the liver and glycogen. And protein supplies additional glucose to the body from glucose breakdown from the liver.

For arterial health: 10-30 grams
-High blood sugar is the leading cause of a heart attack. It is the leading cause of blindness, limb amputation, kidney failure, and impotence. This arterial disease results from widespread glycation (sugar coating) from high blood sugar. Over the course of the day, whether we drip 150 grams of sugar slowly or quickly, into arteries (as fat cells) the damage is the same. Fiber can limit blood sugar spikes, but does not reduce high blood sugar levels. All the fiber in the world cannot prevent 150 grams of carbohydrate from eventually hitting the bloodstream. A low grain and fruit diet is the most ideal diet for someone who wants to live to be 120.   10 grams a day is more than sufficient for individuals taking insulin with type 1 diabetes. It is more than sufficient for the average American looking for ideal health.

For mental health: 10-30 grams
-Only red blood cells, reproductive organs, and cancer cells run on sugar metabolism. The rest of the body generates its energy from fat. Low carbohydrate diets are known to reverse symptoms of epilepsy, prevent dementia and Alzheimers. When one has 10 grams a day of carbohydrate, the need for sleep is closer to six hours. On 50 grams a day, the need for sleep approaches 8 hours. Blood sugar is not raised by carbohydrate, but lowered due to insulin release. More stable levels of glucose are provided by protein breakdown in the liver. For ideal sleep, mood, mental health, and happiness, 10 grams a day is ideal.

For spiritual health: 10-30 grams a day
-When we eat fast food, burgers, hot dogs, and cheese, we pollute our bodies and our souls. When we harm the environment and mistreat our animals, we harm our health and our human spirit. Many of the emotional disorders we suffer have their roots in overeating and improper nutrition. One cannot acquire wisdom when one is hungry or ill. A small hole in the body creates a larger hole in the soul. In general, following the middle path is the wisest one. But as with everything in nature, to everything there is a season. We must have the humility to learn from Nature and wildlife. Joy and gladness increase our ability to reach our health and life goals. The more joyful we are, the more we are able to overcome our obstacles rather than go under them.

For Cancer: 10-30 grams a day
-Insulin is widely considered the single leading food based cause of cancer today, above aflatoxin and food additives. Individuals with Diabetes are roughly 30 per cent more likely to develop colorectal cancer. Women with diabetes have a 20 per cent greater risk of developing breast cancer. People with diabetes had an 82 per cent higher risk of developing pancreatic cancer Insulin is expressed six to eight times the amount on cancer cells as normal cells. The lower the carbohydrate in the diet, the less the risk of breast cancer and other cancers.

For Athletes: 10-30 grams a day
-Today, we are no longer hunter-gatherers. A 40-30-30 diet is irrelevant. Today, we are no longer active 5am in the morning to 5pm at night day laborers and field workers. Exercise is ultimately what helps us lose body fat. Losing weight through diet alone is extremely difficult. 10 grams a day is an absolute maximum for the average sedentary person. Insulin is the powerful lock and key for body fat. A low insulin promoting diet will help a person untap greater potential from exercise.
-An agrarian diet without exercise is the major cause of obesity and diabetes. They are rare in nomadic, hunter-gatherer, and island nations.

The National Weight Control Registry (NWCR) is a registry of more than 2000 individuals who have lost more than 30 pounds and maintained their weight for one year. The Registry shows that the two most important aspects were exercise of at least 60 minutes a day, and a consistent dietary regimen with less variety of food choices, and at least one meal in which the same food was always eaten. 75% reported eating breakfast. Such factors as a methodical, disciplined diet, structure and routine were the factors that played the largest role along with exercise. A plan, timetable, and calendar, and regular meal plan regiment, therefore, may be the most helpful, for losing weight. Most say that they kept the weight off by eating right and exercising 60 to 90 minutes a day. In order to maintain their weight after 30 pounds, most users in the registry had to exercise between 60 to 90 minutes a day to maintain the weight loss.

For Weight loss: 10-30 grams
-The body cannot make fat from fat. Calories do not make a person fat. Only sugar is the element that makes the body fat. 1000 calories from fat cannot create body fat. 10,000 fat calories cannot create a drop of fat in fat cells. 100,000 calories from fat in the diet cannot create fat in fat cells. Only a sugar molecule makes body fat and makes fat in the liver.
- All the sugar required for the body is provided by protein in the diet. No carbohydrate is required for life. Protein in the diet provides the blood sugar needs of all carnivores, whether a cat, dog, sea mammal, primate, or human being. Nothing in the ocean eats fruit and cereal. No carnivore eats fruit and cereal. Our government tells us cereal and fruit should represent 90% of our diet. There are no essential carbohydrates in the diet. These are the two food groups least required for life. All carnivores attest to this fact.
-The amount required to inhibit "ketosis" or weight loss, is 10 grams of carbohydrate for an average resting human. It is roughly 50 grams for someone exercising. Any more than 10 grams a day for someone not exercising may lead to slow weight gain. After 30 years of slow weight gain, it is easily understandable how one in three American men are obese, and one in two women. 10 grams a day is a very reasonable diet for both every day health and long-term health. The closer one can get to 10 grams a day in the diet, largely from legumes, vegetables, and seeds, nuts, and oils, the more one will lose weight.
- The average bowl of cereal has as much carbohydrate as one to two chocolate bars. Few grains are low in starch with the exception of fiber supplements or cereals marketed as 60-70% fiber. Even whole grain oats, barley, and rye are 88% starch and less than 12% fiber. Other cereals are less than 5% fiber. In the typical oat cereal, 28 grams come from starch and less than 4 from fiber. Some rare fruits such as raspberries and lemons are low in sugar. Low sugar cereal grains are not oats, barley, and rye, but specialty high fiber cereals that remove 90% of the starch component. Popular culture perceives fruit juice as healthy and high in Vitamin C. Studies now show sugar fruit juice is as high in sugar as coca

cola. The findings show orange juice is as likely to cause diabetes. By logic, it is also as likely to lead to obesity as a coca cola. Fruit juices often contain 50-80 grams per glass, almost three candy bars. A teaspoon of table sugar has only 4 grams of carbohydrate, compared to 80 in a glass of grape juice. Fruit sugar or fructose is four to five times more likely to glue itself to an artery than glucose, which is the digested component of all starch. A bowl of Sucrose, a mixture of table glucose and fructose produces lower blood sugar levels and insulin levels than a bowl of crystalline starch, or pure glucose on digestion. Fruit juices, cereal grain, and bread, the most consumed foods in America, are the leading cause of Obesity and Diabetes. The typical American breakfast poses the single greatest risk to one's health. The current average intake of Americans is 150 grams of carbohydrate a day, the equivalent of five chocolate bars of sugar.

Fuel use of Muscle by Sport

Rest, fasting	fatty acids, no glucose
Low intensity	fatty acid, limited use of glycogen, no glucose
Marathon	fatty acids, limited use of glycogen, no glucose
Sprinting	glycogen, glucose

The Body uses fat for fuel. Only Red blood cells and Cancer cells use sugar for fuel. Carbohydrate loading is a myth. It is not recommended for exercise and causes rapid low blood sugar after insulin responds, known as "hitting the wall" to the runner which coincides with weakness, shaking,even fainting.

Typical Meals

Breakfast:
Fish—wild Pacific salmon, sardine, or cod (high omega 3)
Water with three squeezed lemons
One slice bread

Lunch:
A fresh sardine or mackerel salad with dark greens, olive oil, vinegar and raspberries
Mushrooms stuffed with veggie cheese, tomato sauce, and garlic
Spinach with veggie cheese, mustard seeds, garlic, curry powder

Dinner:
Tofu with garlic, ginger, chopped tomato and soy sauce
Spinach Salad with grapefruit and vinaigrette
Cream of Cauliflower Soup

Healthy Snacks

Vegetables:
Falafel with veggies and hummus
Ratatouille or Eggplant parmagiana
Avocado and tomato salad

Nuts:
Sesame seed butter
Pumpkin butter
Roasted Chestnuts

Fruit:
Bowl of Raspberries
Half grapefruit
Half an apple

Grain:
F-factor cereal with berries and Coconut milk (unless gluten intolerant)

Drinks:
Homemade lemonade with 2 teaspoons sugar
Coconut milk
Coconut water
Miso soup

Protein:
Hangar steak sandwich on half a roll
Salmon tempura
Bison burger on half a roll

"There are times when a critic truly risks something, and that is in the discovery and defense of the "new." The world is often unkind to new talent, new creations. The new needs friends. Last night, I experienced something new: a... meal from a singularly unexpected source. To say that both the meal and its maker have challenged my preconceptions about fine cooking is a gross understatement. They have rocked me to my core. In the past, I have made no secret of my disdain for Chef Gusteau's famous motto, "Anyone can cook." But I realize, only now do I truly understand what he meant. Not everyone can become a great artist; but a great artist can come from anywhere. It is difficult to imagine more humble origins than those...now cooking at Gusteau's."

-From the Children's Movie "Ratatouille"

Recipes

Soup:
Fish soup
Persian soup
Cauliflower soup
Cream of asparagus soup
Cream of mushroom soup
Lentil Soup

Vegetables:
Mashed garlic cauliflower
Vegetable masala
Cream of spinach
Stuffed artichoke hearts in garlic sauce
Black eyed peas
Mustard Greens
Falafel
Vegetable Tagine
Greens with vinaigrette dressing
Fried Tofu in Garlic sauce
Ratatouille

Fish:
Fried fish with garlic aioli sauce
Sole meuniere
Curried salmon
Salmon in rice paper
Fresh Sardines in olive oil

Chicken:
Tandoori Chicken
Chicken Tikka
Chicken Korma
Moroccan Chicken
Yemen Chicken

Israeli Chicken
Chicken Paprika
Orange Chicken
Ethiopian Chicken

Meat: (lean, grass-fed organic only)
Garlic Lamb
Skirt Steak au Poivre
Skirt Steak Madeira

Vegetable Side Dishes and Dips:
Ginger Paste
Green Masala
Harissa
Spiced butter
Za'Atar
Hummus
Ginger Chutney with beets
Chili Lime Mayonaisse
Piri Piri
Peach Barbeque Sauce
Satay
Roasted Garlic
Chermoula
White Bean Puree

Cooking Directions for All Dishes

Take all spices, organic oil (preferably organic coconut), garlic, onion, and herbs (chives, dill, parsley) a touch of sugar, salt, fresh lemon and pepper to taste and simmer in oil a few minutes until browned. Typically the more garlic, the better.

Add fish, meat, or poultry into large pan or 2 large pans as needed and sauté until golden brown and three quarters cooked

Add base sauce of tomatoes, wine, beef or chicken stock, or coconut cream as sauce recommends into pan. Chicken or beef stock can be added to most all of these dishes.

Simmer on low heat and stir occasionally until fully cooked. I have prepared these recipes many times and rarely has it mattered how many spices I've added. The only one to watch is too much salt or soy sauce, sugar, vinegar, or cayenne, or tomato paste if one is not using fresh tomato. Typically too much garlic, onion, fresh tomato, pepper, coconut cream, wine or curry rarely ruins a dish.

Since fat doesn't make us fat, it is perfectly reasonable to sauté all dishes. And for batter, one can use crushed almonds instead of flour. If flour is desired, this is much lower in carbohydrate to batter chicken or fish than eat a bowl of pasta, potatoes, or other high carbohydrate rich meal. A few ounces of flour will not significantly increase the carbohydrate content of the meal, so breading any entrée is reasonable.

Once you become used to sautéing most dishes, cooking becomes easy, and even a little wine and soy sauce takes just minutes to prepare. (see Israeli Chicken Schnitzel). Indian sauces may take longer.

Coconut cream is much preferred to coconut milk to thicken sauces. If this is difficult to find, one can refrigerate coconut milk and skim off the cream. Tofu cream cheese or cheeses can be used in place of dairy cheese.

Prepared curry spice mixes are relatively easy to find. When available, use fresh organic vegetables and herbs, and refrigerate herbs and even spices to keep them fresh. When shopping in the market, keep in mind "protein" and "vegetables" and this will simplify your shopping list so you may not even need to make a list of ingredients. Stick to the outside aisles, usually fresh fish and produce. The inner aisles are usually processed carbohydrates.

Meat is best left out of refrigerator 2 hours at room temperature before cooking.

Fish Soup

6 cloves garlic
2 tsp salt
7 cup water
2 to 3 pound fish (salmon, cod, halibut)
Quarter cup olive oil
3 tbsp parsley
One and half cup dry white wine
1 tsp saffron
2 cups tomato
1 bay leaf
Half tsp thyme
1 tbsp basil
2 tbsp zest from orange peel
2 onions

Add ingredients to bowl and simmer 30 minutes
or until ready

Persian Soup

1/2kg of diced meat boiled in water
1 big chopped onion
red/white beans (half cooked)
chopped vegetables
3 sundried lemons (Persian specialty)
washed and shred into small pieces
1/2 teaspoon of cumin
1/2 teaspoon of black pepper
1 spoon of chicken stock
a pinch of salt

To prepare the previous night:

Soak the red (or white) beans in water all
night and rinse off the next day with cold
water
Chop de following vegetables very small:
spinach, beet leaves, coriander and some
celery leaves (you can prepare a bigger
amount and save in the freezer)

Fry the onion in a bit of oil, add the meat and stir.
Add the red beans to the meat. When the meat is
half cooked, add boiling water up to half the pan
together with the chopped vegetables, sliced
lemons and spices. Stir.

Cauliflower Soup

3 tbsp veg oil
1 garlic clove
3 cups cauliflower
1 cup chicken broth
1 cup cream substitute (Soya (tofu) cream)
1 bay leaf
2 tsp rosemary
2 tbsp lime

Add ingredients and simmer 20 to 30 minutes until soft
Do not boil
Then puree

Cream of Asparagus Soup

2 tbsp margarine
3 pound asparagus
4 cup chicken broth
Juice half lemon
Half cup nondairy creamer (Soya (tofu) cream)
Sautee veggies
Add veg broth
Add cream and lemon juice

Cream of Mushroom Soup

7 cups low sodium chicken broth or fresh chicken
soup
4 cloves garlic
2 pounds mushrooms
2 shallots
2 parsley sprigs
1 tsp rosemary
3 garlic cloves
3 sprigs thyme
One and half tsp salt
Quarter tsp pepper
5 tbsp margarine
Half cup cream substitute (Soya (tofu) cream)

Add ingredients to large saucepan and stir
Add mushrooms
Stir frequently 20 to 30 minutes
Remove sprigs of parsley and thyme
Do not boil

Lentil Soup

2 cups lentils
3 garlic cloves
5 tablespoons margarine
5 cups water
Juice half lemon
Half tsp salt
1 tsp sugar
1 tsp oregano
Half teaspoon cumin
3 cloves
1 cinnamon stick

Simmer in large pot
Add margarine

Garlic Mashed Cauliflower

2 pounds cauliflower
8 cloves garlic
1 cup low salt chicken broth
half cup of water
2 tsp salt
10 tbsp non dairy cream substitute (soya (tofu) cream)
6 tsp oil (avocado, apricot seed, canola, and macadamia)
Boil in lg pot
Add soy and oil
Blend and serve in casserole

Vegetable Masala

1 cup chickpeas
1 quart water
Half cup asparagus
Half head chopped cauliflower
1 tsp salt
2 tbsp canola
1 tsp mustard seed
1 tsp cumin
1 onion chopped
2 tomatoes chopped
1 tsp garam masala
half tsp ginger
4 cloves garlic chopped finely
half tsp pepper
3 tbsp parsley

Heat oil and cook mustard seeds, cumin, add onion and garlic and sauté. Stir in tomatoes, garam masala, ginger, garlic, salt, pepper. Sauté. Add cooked vegetables to tomato mixture and sauté a few minutes.

Cream of Spinach

2 frozen spinach thawed or 3 cans chopped
spinach
Boil and drain spinach
Add to pot:
3 tbsp oil (canola, apricot kernel, macadamia)
2 bay leaf
3 garlic cloves
Whisk in 1 and half cup cream substitute) (soya
(tofu) cream
Add spinach
Touch of salt and pepper

Stuffed Artichoke Hearts with Tomato Sauce

6 artichoke hearts
Chop 7 mushrooms, cook in olive oil until soft
and then dice, drain and set aside
Prepare tomato sauce:

1 tbsp olive oil
4 garlic cloves
1 can tomatoes drained and chopped or 1 pound
tomatoes seeded and chopped
1 tsp sugar
1 tablespoon lemon juice
1 cup water
Half teaspoon thyme
2 tablespoons parsley
1 tsp coriander

Fill inside of artichoke hearts with mushrooms
Pour sauce over
Spice with red pepper flakes

Alternate: Stuff mushroom caps with soy cheese
and garlic tomato sauce

Black Eyed Peas

1 cup black eyed peas
5 tbsp oil
3 tomatoes
4 garlic cloves chopped
one inch ginger piece chopped
1 tsp pepper
1 cup coconut milk
1 tsp paprika
1 cup chicken stock
1 tsp salt
2 cilantro sprigs

combine peas with 4 cups water and simmer 45
minutes
add garlic, ginger and sauté 10 minutes
add tomato, coconut milk, chicken stock, and
cilantro
and simmer until thick

Mustard Greens

6 cups mustard greens
4 tbsp oil
6 garlic cloves
3 inches ginger peeled and chopped
1 tbsp mustard seeds
1 tsp lemongrass
2 and half cups chicken stock
1 tsp salt

Bring pot of salted water to boil. Add mustard greens, blanch for 30 seconds and transfer to plate and drain.

Add ingredients and sauté in oil

add to pot, bring to simmer for 10 minutes

Fold in mustard greens and cook 2 minutes. Season with the salt.

Falafel

1 cup dried chickpeas soaked in cold water one day
and drained
5 garlic cloves, crushed
2 tsp ground coriander
1/4 tsp ginger
1 tsp pepper
quarter cup chopped parsley
2 tsp salt
½ tsp baking soda
2 tablespoon lemon juice
3 cups oil for deep frying

Combine ingredients and chop until fine. Add 1
tbsp coconut milk.

Heat 3 inches oil in deep pot over medium heat.

Scoop balls into oil, frying until golden brown, 3 to
5 minutes

serve with hummus, tahini, vegetables, fried
eggplant

Vegetable Tagine

Half head cauliflower, peeled and cut into 1 inch
cubes
half cup canola oil
2 eggplants sliced thinly
1 onion, cut into half inch pieces
5 garlic cloves chopped
Quarter cup olives, halved and pitted
2 tsp tandoori powder
2 cups vegetable stock
2 tsp salt
1 tsp pepper
2 tbsp parsley chopped
3 prunes, unpitted
3 apricots, unpitted

Boil beets, drain and set aside

Heat oil and add ingredients sautéing until
eggplant tender
about 10 mins with onion and garlic, and olives

Stir in other ingredients

Simmer 20 mins

stir in parsley

Salad Greens with Vinaigrette

2 lemons
4 tbs red wine vinegar
4 tbsp Dijon
1 cup virgin olive oil
Half tsp salt
Quarter tsp pepper

Fried Tofu in Garlic Sauce

1 box firm tofu
1 egg
¾ cup cornstarch
Canola oil
2 chopped onions
1 tbsp ground fresh ginger
3 tbsp ground fresh garlic
½ cup vegetable stock
2 tsp soy sauce
4 tbsp sugar
1 tbsp vinegar
Pinch Red pepper flakes

Freeze tofu night before and drain
Cut into one inch pieces
Mix egg with three tablespoons water and dip tofu in mixture
Cover tofu in cornstarch
Fry tofu until brown and set aside
Drain oil
Heat three tbsp canola and add onions, garlic and ginger and cook until lightly browned
Add other ingredients (stock, soy sauce, vinegar, sugar, and pinch of red pepper flakes)
Mix 1 tbsp cornstarch and 2 tbsp water and add this to mixture
Add fried tofu, stir, and serve

Ratatouille

2 Japanese (soft purple) medium size eggplants
3 Fresh vine tomatoes
2 peppers
1 red onion
5 cloves garlic
2 tablespoons miso paste
2 tbsp soy sauce
1 tbsp sweet white wine
½ cup dry white wine
1 tbsp brown sugar
¼ cup Canola oil
¾ cup water
2 tsp pepper

Slice eggplant into thin round strips
Put water and salt into big bowl and soak eggplant
inside for 30 mins to eliminate bitter taste, drain,
and towel dry
Put oil, and garlic into pan and heat until bubbling
Add eggplant and sauté until soft
Add onion and peppers and tomatoes and stir
Add dry wine, miso paste, brown sugar and water
and simmer until liquid reduced 50% for 25
minutes
Add soy sauce, sweet wine and simmer 3 minutes
Serve with chopped scallions and add soy sauce to
taste

Fried fish with Garlic Aioli

2 pound haddock or cod

Marinade:
Quarter cup white wine vinegar
5 garlic cloves
Tbsp parsley
3 tbsp lemon juice
1 tbsp olive oil
Half tsp thyme

Batter in:
1 egg
half cup flour
half cup rice flour
tsp salt
tsp b. powder
1 bottle cold beer
Fry in 4 cups canola

Garlic aioli:
Three quarter cups mayo
6 garlic cloves
Tsp sugar
Quarter Tsp salt
Quarter cup fresh lemon juice

Sole Meuniere

4 fillets
All purpose flour for frying
2 tbsp capers
1 med lemon
2 garlic cloves
7 tbsp canola, apricot kernel, avocado or
macadamia oil
Third cup water
2 tbsp non dairy creamer (soya (tofu) cream)
3 tbsp sherry vinegar
1 tsp salt
1 tsp pepper
Dip fish in flour, fry and remove
Sautee additional ingredients
add capers and juice of lemon
spread over fish

Curried Salmon

2 pound salmon
1 tsp cumin
5 garlic cloves
1 cup water
1 tsp tamarind paste
2 tomatoes
1 tbsp br sugar
1 tsp cilantro
1 tsp coriander
Pinch cinnamon
Quarter tsp cardamom
Half tsp cayenne
1 lg onion
3 tbsp canola or avocado oil

Sautee spices in oil
Cook fish in oil until browned
Add tomatoes, tamarind, sugar, water, and simmer
on low flame until cooked

Salmon in Rice Paper

4 3 oz fillets
Juice 1 lime
2 inches ginger grated
2 tbs cilantro fish
4 scallions chopped
1 garlic cloves crushed
8 rice paper wrappers
Quarter cup sunflower oil

Mix together ingredients and sprinkle over salmon
Soak rice paper 15 secs
Remove water

Place fish on each
Fold to enclose fish
Heat oil in frying pan
Add and fry until rice paper golden 5 to 10 mins
and fish tender
Drizzle with choice of sauce, dip

Fried Sardines in Olive Oil

10 fresh sardines
¾ cup extra virgin olive oil
5 garlic cloves, minced
4 tbsp fresh parsley

Debone spine and remove gut of fish with sharp
knife
Bread in tempura or similar batter
Cook in olive oil until cooked 1 minute each side
Transfer to a dish
Cook garlic until almost brown
Add parsley and stir 30 seconds
Pour over sardines and serve with bread

Tandoori Chicken

10 chicken thighs skin removed
Half cup sour supreme
3 tbsp non dairy creamer (soy (tofu) cream)
4 garlic cloves
1 tsp chili powder
Juice 2 lemons
Half inch ginger root
1 tsp cilantro
1 tsp coriander
2 tsp paprika
Half cup tomato sauce
Make sauce of ingredients
Marinate chicken overnight
Then cook in tin foil with spices, serve with lemon

Chicken Tikka

6 chicken thighs
One can low sodium chicken broth or soup
5 fresh high quality tomatoes
canola oil to coat pan
7 cloves garlic
3 tsp cumin
1 tsp coriander
1 tsp cinnamon
2 tsp pepper
1 tbsp ground ginger fresh
4 tsp salt
2 tsp paprika
1 tbsp fresh ground parsley
Quarter cup chopped fresh cilantro
Juice half lemon
One can coconut cream (or coconut milk)
One cup sour supreme
Sautee spices and garlic
Cook chicken in spices until browned
Drain extra oil from pan
Add tomatoes, broth and coconut cream, cover
and let simmer

Chicken Korma

3 pound chicken
One can low sodium chicken broth or soup
Two third cup margarine
7 cloves garlic
1 tsp coriander
1 tbsp cinnamon
1 tsp cloves
1 tbsp parsley
1 tsp cardamom
Juice half lemon
One cup soya (tofu) cream or sour supreme

Sautee spices and garlic
Cook chicken in spices until browned
Drain additional oil from pan
Add broth, cream cover and let simmer

Moroccan Chicken

12 chicken thigh
3 cloves garlic
3 tbsp thyme
1 tbsp cumin
2 tsp ginger
1 tbsp salt
1 cup red wine
3 tsp pepper
Half cup br sugar
Zest 3 lemons
2 tsp cinnamon
2 tsp cilantro
7 figs
1 cup chicken soup low salt
Quarter cup ground walnuts
3 tbsp macadamia or apricot kernel oil

Sautee spices in oil
Cook meat in oil until browned
Add figs, chicken broth, wine and simmer on low
flame until cooked

Yemen Chicken

12 chicken thigh
12 cloves garlic
1 tsp pepper
Pinch chili powder
3 tbsp margarine
1 tbsp cumin
1 tbsp cilantro
1 tsp paprika
2 cups chicken soup low salt
2 tbsp lemon juice

Sautee spices in oil
Cook meat in oil until browned
Add broth and simmer on low flame until cooked

Israeli Chicken

6 chicken thighs
2 tsp soy sauce
1/2 tsp pepper
2 tsp fresh lemon
2 tsp sugar
2 tbsp parsley
Half cup rose wine
Quarter to half cup unsweetened almond milk
Serves three

Breading for chicken thighs:
Half cup canola oil
4 tablespoons tahini
1 whole chopped onion
2 tbsp Sage and rosemary
Stir ingredients
Spread paste over top chicken
Dip in corn flake crumbs
Repeat
Fry chicken in canola oil until brown

Then prepare wine sauce, add to fried chicken in
pan and reduce thirty minutes over low heat.

Chicken Paprika

3 pound chicken
3 tbsp canola oil
4 cloves garlic
4 tomatoes
Half cup sour supreme (sour cream substitute)
1 cup chicken broth
3 tsp paprika

Sautee spices in oil
Cook meat in oil until browned
Add tomatoes, broth, cream and simmer on low
flame until cooked

Orange Chicken

10 chicken thigh
Juice 2 oranges
2 tsp pepper
3 tbsp apricot kernel, macadamia oil, or canola
1 cup chicken broth
1 tsp tarragon
2 tbsp coriander
2 tbsp brown sugar
2 tbsp parsley
1 shallot
1 garlic clove
Quarter cup white or rose wine (optional)

Sautee spices in oil
Cook meat in oil until browned
Add broth, wine, juice, sugar, and simmer on low
flame until cooked

Ethiopian Chicken

2 med onions
Salt
4 tbsp margarine salted
quarter tsp cardamom
half tsp black pepper
3 cloves
2 garlic cloves
1 and half inch piece ginger chipped
1 tbsp beriberi or chili powder
2 and half cups chicken stock, divided
4 to 5 pounds chicken
half cup dry red wine
juice of lime
2 hard boiled eggs peeled

combine onions, pinch salt, and half margarine in
large deep pot over low heat
Stir until onions golden about 15 mins
Add remaining margarine, cardamom, pepper,
cloves, garlic, ginger and beriberi
cook 10 mins

Add 2 cups chicken stock and chicken
simmer
gently stir in lime juice and eggs and simmer 5
mins

Garlic Lamb

10 large cloves garlic
three sprigs fresh rosemary
¼ cup olive oil
Salt and fresh pepper
7 lamb chops
1 tbsp vinegar
2 oozes. teriyaki marinade sauce
1 tsp Worcestershire sauce
4 oz. white wine
3 tbsp chopped mint
1 tbsp. fresh parsley, chopped
1 oz. brandy
3/4 stick margarine
serve with chopped parsley

mix teriyaki, Worcestershire and wine. Marinate.

Place the garlic and rosemary and olive oil and
mint, chop until a paste is made and press paste
firmly onto surface of lamb chops. Cook lamb in
oil.

Bring marinade to boil and serve over lamb

Steak au Poivre

2 tbsp whole peppercorns
4 hangar (Skirt) steaks
2 tbsp canola oil
¼ cup cognac or brandy
1 cup beef stock
4 tbsp margarine unsalted
1 cup coconut cream

Remove steak from fridge an hour before cooking
Crush peppercorns and place evenly over steak on
both sides of steak on a plate
Sautee steaks in oil and margarine and cook until
done and place aside
Add cognac to pan pouring off excess fat but not
all fat
Carefully ignite alcohol with long match
Shake pan until flames die
Return pan to medium heat
Add stock and coconut cream and cook until
reduced in half so thick
Add steak back to pan to heat
Serve

Steak Madeira Sauce

(4 steaks)
Quarter cup canola or apricot kernel oil
Tsp tarragon
Half bay leaf
2 tbsp parsley
2 shallots
Three quarter cup red wine
2 and half cup beef broth
Quarter cup sherry or brandy w tsp cornstarch

Sautee spices in oil
Cook meat in oil until browned
Add wine and simmer on low flame until cooked

Ginger Paste

3 garlic cloves minced
2 tbs ginger ground
1 tsp coriander
half tsp pepper
3 tbsp tahini (ground sesame)
third cup lemon juice
half tsp salt

heat garlic, ginger, coriander, tahini, and brown 2 minutes in sauce pan

Transfer to food processor.

Add oil, lemon juice and process.

Green Masala

2 inch piece ginger grated
5 garlic cloves minced
5 jalapenos chopped seeds removed
4 black cloves
half tsp cardamom seeds
2 oz mint leaves chopped
1 oz cilantro leaves chopped
1 tsp cinnamon
Quarter cup cider vinegar
1 tsp salt
¼ cup sesame oil
¼ cup sunflower or canola oil
1 tsp fenugreek seeds

heat quarter cup sunflower oil and quarter cup
sesame oil
add garlic, ginger, spices and jalapenos and sauté 4
mins

stir in vinegar and blend

Harissa

5 ounces chili peppers, seeds removed
half cup virgin olive oil
7 garlic cloves peeled
1 tsp cumin
1 tsp coriander
1 tsp salt
1 tbsp mint
quarter cup fresh cilantro

Soak peppers in warm water until soft
Squeeze out excess water
Process peppers in food processor
heat oil, add garlic and sauté spices
add ingredients to peppers and blend to thick red
puree
let sit for a few days before serving
use in moderation as is very spicy

Spiced Butter

1 pound margarine
half medium red onion
1 garlic clove minced
one 3 inch piece ginger finely chopped
1 tsp fenugreek seeds
1 tsp cumin
1 tsp cardamom seeds
1 tsp dried oregano
half tsp turmeric
8 basil leaves

melt margarine on low heat
add ingredients and stir 15 minutes

Za'atar

2 tbsp sesame seeds
2 tbsp thyme
1 tbsp oregano
¼ cup sumac
1 tsp salt

toast sesame seeds on low heat 2 mins
mix rest of ingredients in bowl and stir in sesame
seeds and salt

store in cool place

Hummus with Roasted Garlic and Pepper

2 cups dried chickpeas soaked in cold water for 7-
8 hours and drained
1 med onion
5 garlic cloves
quarter cup olive oil
1 chili seeds removed
1 tsp Harissa

combine chickpeas and onion in sauce pan, add 4
cups water, and boil

Reduce heat and simmer one and half hour

drain, reserving cup of cooking liquid

Preheat oven to 325F

Add chilies and garlic to pan 10 mins

Add roasted garlic, and chili, chickpeas, harissa,
and remaining 2 tbsp oil
and 3 tbsp reserved cooking liquid

Puree

Ginger Chutney with Beets

2 tbsp olive oil
2 cups red onions diced
4 garlic cloves minced
3 two inch pieces ginger, peeled and sliced
3 beets
1 tbsp honey
3 cardamom pods
2 thyme sprigs
2 tbsp sugar
2 tbsp raisins
1 tbsp margarine
Half cup water
Quarter cup red wine vinegar
half tsp salt

Heat oil
Add onions, garlic, ginger and beets
sauté 15 mins

Add honey, cardamom, thyme, sugar, vinegar,
raisins, butter and stir 1 minute

add chicken stock and simmer 40 mins until beets
are soft

remove cardamom, thyme and ginger from the
chutney, and stir in the salt.

Chili Lime Mayonnaise

1 cup olive oil
1 tbsp almonds
2 garlic cloves
1/2 tsp chili powder
2 tbsp cilantro
3 egg yolks
quarter cup fresh lime juice
2 tsp red wine vinegar
¾ cup canola
salt and pepper

heat tbsp olive oil in sauté pan
add almonds and garlic and stir until brown 3 mins
add chilies, chili powder, and cook 2 mins until
soft

transfer to blender, add egg yolks and blend well

add oil in thin steady stream

season with salt and pepper

Piri Piri

7 red chilies, chopped, seeds removed
Quarter cup fresh lemon juice
3 tbsp fresh cilantro chopped
1 tbsp parsley chopped
1 tbsp paprika
3 garlic cloves
1 tsp salt
Half cup olive oil

combine chilies, lemon juice, cilantro, parsley, paprika, salt and garlic in blender

add oil in slow stream and blend

Barbeque Sauce

2 tbsp coconut oil
1 med red onion diced
6 tomatoes, seeded and chipped
three inch piece ginger grated
13 garlic cloves minced
1 chili finely chopped
2 cups water
quarter cup brewed decaf coffee
2 tsp chili powder
tsp mustard
quarter tsp coriander seeds crushed
quarter cup honey
half cup cider vinegar
1 tsp cinnamon
1 chopped peach and quarter cup fresh lemon
juice blended)

heat oil in large saucepan over high heat
add ingredients and simmer 40 mins on reduced
heat
add honey and simmer 10 mins

Satay

1 tbsp ground ginger
1/3 cup coconut cream or milk
1 and half tsp cayenne pepper
3 garlic cloves minced
1 cup peanut oil
2 tbsp soy sauce
2 tbsp brown sugar

Add to sauté pan all but oil over medium heat and toast for one minute

Transfer to blender and stir in oil.

Roasted Garlic

10 heads garlic
5 tbsp olive oil

cut off top head garlic head
preheat oven to 375
place garlic on foil and sprinkle peanut oil
wrap foil around garlic and place on baking sheet
roast 35 to 45 mins until garlic is soft

squeeze garlic from skin or eat whole

Chermoula

½ tsp coriander seeds
10 black peppercorns
½ tsp salt
1 tsp paprika
1 medium onion
1/3 cup fresh parsley
2 tbsp lemon juice
2 tbsp lemon peel
2 tbsp olive oil
2 tbsp fresh coriander
4 garlic cloves chopped
2 tsp ginger

Serve with fish

Roasted Garlic White Bean Puree

1 cup dried white cannelloni beans
3 tbsp olive oil
juice of 1 lemon
1 tbsp sage
1 tbsp rosemary
salt and pepper
1 cup veggie or chicken stock

combine beans in bowl or pot and soak overnight
Drain beans and place in pan with water, stock, and spices and bring to boil
Simmer gently uncovered 1 hour or until beans soft
Transfer beans to processor with 2 bulbs roasted garlic (see recipe) reserving some of cooking liquid
Add remaining lemon juice and oil and add some of reserved cooking liquid to desired consistency.

Remedies from Nature

Adrenal:
Vitamin C
Lecithin--- sunflower seeds

Allergies:
Vitamin C
Garlic
Wheatgrass
Chlorophyll
Ant parasite
Antiviral--- Ginger
Bioflavanoids
Nettle—less—hormonal issues

Alzheimer's:
Reduced carbohydrate consumption
Omega Three from fish oil or seaweed
Sunflower seed butter--- for lecithin- phosphatidyl choline
and serine

Anemia:
Greens formula--- i.e. Wheatgrass, barleygrass,alfalfa,etc.
for B vitamins and iron
B12--- molasses, biostrath (lozenges), non-live brewer's
yeast
Folic acid--- leafy vegetables
Iron--- lentils, salmon, meat
iron

Anorexia:
Zinc--- sea vegetables, seafood
Copper
Ginger
Coconut oil--- easily absorbed

Anxiety:
Magnesium or Greens powder (rich in magnesium)
B-12

L-theanine
Taurine
Vitamin C

Appendicitis:
Antibiotic
probiotic
Wheatgrass
Chlorophyll

Arteries:
Vitamin C--- clears calcium deposits from high blood sugar
Omega three--- vasodilator
Horse chestnut
Butchers broom
Grapeseed extract
resveratrol

Arthritis:
Omega 3s (fish oil)
Garlic—antibacterial
Ginger-- antiviral
Probiotic—antibacterial--- acidophilus
Cranberry
Myrrh
Avoidance of lectins--- eggplant, potato, peppers

Asthma:
Fish oil
Liver cleanse
Greens formula – wheatgrass, barley grass, etc.

Athlete's foot:
Coconut oil
Caprilic acid- from coconut
Ginger—enzymes
Oregano
Oil of myrrh or oregano applied to foot

Attention deficit:
DHA--- fish oil derivative
EPA--- fish oil derivative (enteric coated better than liquid)
Or EFas (essential fatty acid formula)
Vitamin C
B-12 lozenges

Autism
Avoid vaccinations pre 1983 (DTP, OPV, MMR) . Since 1983, the number of vaccines has gone from 10 to 36. Autism has gone from 1 in 10000 in 1983 to 1 in 150 in 2008. Lawsuits of 28 billion dollars have already been awarded due to tainted vaccines. Nevertheless, the total number of vaccines may also play the major role in inflammatory disorders and neurological impairment.

Autoimmune (lupus, MS, vasculitis):
GI cleanse (see Crohns)-- GI is large area of immune activity
Antiviral (ginger or digestive enzyme formula)
Ant parasitic (see parasite) - black walnut, cloves, Artemisia)
Liver cleanse
Kidney cleanse
Heavy metal detoxification
Blood type specific diet (in addition to low carbohydrate) especially for type AB blood
Low carbohydrate diet--- glycosylation of arteries causes immune response to arteries
Removal of all but emergency medication (inhaler, antibiotic for severe infection)
Avoidance of antibiotics
Probiotic--- prevents build-up of mycobacteria and klebsiella which make GI permeable
No dairy, soy, gluten in diet

Bacterial infection:
Garlic
Oregano
Probiotics-- (antibacterial)
Ginger
Chlorella (Nature's peroxide)
Astragulus
Myrrh
Elderberry
Vitamin C
Omega 3
Ginger
low carbohydrate intake
Maitake mushroom

Bloating:
Acidophilus
Ginger
Avoidance of dairy
Gluten free breads
More vegetarian protein

Blood Pressure:
K—opposes sodium entry into cells
Lower blood sugar levels—lowers insulin which regulates
water balance
Wheatgrass or Barley Grass—high in magnesium
Taurine--- helps support heart muscle contraction
L-carnitine L-tartrate-- assists in muscle cell function
Parsley-- diuretic
Cinnamon—lowers insulin
Chromium—lowers insulin
berberine sulfate-- blood flow

Breast:
Lower insulin levels through diet
See parasite if parasitic or viral origin
Indoles--- Cruciferous vegetables
Calcium d-glucarate
See cancer

Bruising:
Vitamin C
Bioflavanoids-Bromelain, White of citrus fruit
Alfalfa

Cadmium toxicity:
Alfalfa
Garlic
Rutin
Lecithin
Zinc

Cancer:
Digestive Enzymes High Dose – i.e. Enzymedica Digest
Gold or Virastop
Parasite detox formula
Liver detox formula
Kidney detox formula
Low insulin diet
Green Super food Blend (Powders)- Lower insulin levels
and carbohydrate intake (potent growth factor)
Vacustatin – angiogenesis inhibitor (Allergy Research
Group- ARG)
Vitamin C—50 g IV or high dose powder Vitamin C
Biomagnetic resonance therapy (google "Varizapper
Graviola
Arteminisin- from Artemesia Annua—inhibits iron uptake,
antiparasitic (ARG))
Immkine--- lactobacillus immune stimulant (ARG)
Ashwaganda
Maitake mushroom
Reitake Mushroom
Aloe Vera
Natokinase (ARG)
Lectin specific blood type diet
Lycopene
Germanium
Omega 3—5,000 mg daily
PSK/PSP
Polyerga

Cruciferous Vegetable whole food formulas derived from garlic, Brussels sprout, scallion, leek cauliflower, cabbage, onion (New Chapter Vitamins)
cell food
Oregano
D3 (2000-25000)

Candidiasis:
(yeast infections or other fungal infection)
Low carbohydrate diet
Caprylic acid
Coconut oil--- source of caprylic acid
Vitamin C- to improve immune system
Acidophilus
Garlic
Bromelain
low carbohydrate (fungus feeds on sugar) – most important to cure
Biotin
Pau D'Arco
Berberine sulfate
Cinnamon bark
Rosemary leaf extract
Zinc

Canker sores:
Probiotics, Acidophilus

Celiac disease:
Probiotics (i.e. Acidophilus) or mixed probiotics
Olive leaf

Chicken pox:
Beta carotene
Vitamin C
Zinc
Ginger

Cholesterol:
Lower insulin levels and carbohydrate intake

Glucose -> Acetyl Coa -> hmg coA with insulin -> cholesterol, triglycerides -> lipoproteins (LDL, HDL)

Chronic fatigue:
Anti-parasite
Anti-viral—ginger
Greens formula
Fish oil
Malic acid
Fibroboost--- Allergy Research Group

Circulatory problems:
Chlorophyll

Cirrhosis:
Avoid alcohol
Fish oil
Probiotics
Garlic
Milk thistle(silymarin)

Common cold:
Ginger
Omega 3s --- fish oil
Maitake, Reishi, Shiitake (beta 1,3 glucan)
Myrrh
Wheatgrass
Vitamin C
Aloe Vera
Probiotics
Ground cloves
garlic

Cold sores:
Lysine
Zinc

Cortisol:
Lecithin

Pantothenic acid

Crohns, Ulcerative Colitis :
iron
Probiotics
omega 3 fatty acids (fish oil or flax oil)
l-glutamine
bromelain
ginger or papain
vitamin K
avoid unboiled dairy
licorice extract (deglycerinized)
slippery elm bark
antiparasitic
Digestive enzymes
Greens drink i.e. Green Vibrance
limited carbohydrate
high dose Vitamin C (10-20g daily-- powdered unbuffered
vitamin C i.e. Nature's Way or Amla C:
Iron
Pro-50—enteric coated, 15 strains
Omega 3

Croup:
Vitamin C
Zinc
Beta carotene
Fish oil
Ginger

Cystic fibrosis:
Proteolytic enzymes
Beta carotenes
Omega 3 fatty acids

Dandruff:
Low carbohydrate intake
Fish oil
Probiotics—for leaky gut syndrome, a cause of psoriasis
Seaweed—iodine rich

Selenium

Dermatitis (or Psoriasis):
Gi detox—for leaky gut syndrome
Probiotic
Garlic-- antibacterial
Betaine hydrochloride
B12
Fish oil
Kelp
See parasite
Ginger or papaya tablets

Diabetes Type II: (also for high blood sugar, obesity)
Cinnamon. A half teaspoon a day can lead to 20%
improvement in blood sugar. Cinnamon has been used for
several thousand years in traditional Ayurvedic and Greco-
European medical systems. Native to in southern tropical
India, the bark of this evergreen tree has three active
components of cinnamon found to have beneficial
biological activity, increasing insulin-dependent glucose
metabolism by roughly 20-fold in vitro (Anderson RA
2004).

Chromium picolinate (least toxic form) (from arginate or
yeast) . Chromium is an essential trace mineral that plays a
significant role in sugar metabolism. It helps lower blood
sugar levels by improving insulin receptor sensitivity. The
richest natural source is red zinger tea, lemongrass, and
juniper berry and brewers' yeast.

Gymnema Sylvestre The leaves have been used for over
2000 years in India. It Improves insulin release and
insulin's affect. When applied to the tongue, it blocks the
sensation of sweetness.   Interestingly, it produces little
effect in individuals with normal blood sugar.

Bitter melon. (Balsam pear or Momordica Charantia)
Contains charantin, more potent than the oral
hypoglycemic drug tolbutamide. 15 grams of bitter melon

extract produces a 50% decrease in after meal blood sugar. (Y. Srivastava et al. 1993)

Alpha lipoic acid.

Other Useful Compounds:

Vanadyl sulfate. Helps activate transport proteins for glucose uptake functioning much like chromium.

Kino tree bark--- rich in epicatechin and pterostilbene, two antioxidant rich flavonoids. India's Office Council of Medical Research shows in one clinical trial that after 12 weeks, blood sugar dropped over 32 points with 93 patients. A second group produced an average drop of nearly 56 points, with no side effects.

Magnesium and Potassium

lowered carbohydrate intake is a natural diuretic, reducing blood pressure. A wheatgrass or green supplement can replace these minerals naturally.

High dose Intravenous, Liposomal or Powdered Whole Food Vitamin C.
Vitamin C or citrate is the single best natural chelator of calcium from arteries. Modern theories suggest that after glycation from sugar, vitamin C deficiency may be the second leading cause of arterial disease and decay.

Plays a role in lowering insulin utilization.

Selenium 2000mcg
Others compounds found to be helpful:
Banaba (L speciosa)
Jambolan fruit
Neem bark
White kidney bean (lagerstroemia speciosa)
Ptercapus marsupium (5% pterostilbene
Tonspora cordifolia (2,5% bitters)

Ocimum sanctum (ursolic acid 2%)
Green tea extract 20 mg (catechins)

Cortisol lowering – soy lecithin (phosphatidyl serine rich
lowers cortisol, an insulin resistant factor)
Metabolic support--- iodine from kelp for thyroid
Antioxidants-- alpha lipoic acid, IV glutathione for cataract,
glaucoma
Neuropathy-- DHA , lecithin, B-12(for neuropathy)
GI detoxification--- to lower bacteria that feed on sugar

Diarrhea:
Garlic
Probiotics (Acidophilus)
Fiber
Activated Charcoal—for food poisoning

Digestion:
Ginger--- 180 times digestive enzymes of papaya
Licorice--- mucilage
Papaya tablets

Diverticulitis:
Garlic
Probiotics
Fiber
Vitamin C
B complex
Ginger
Alfalfa

Dog bite:
Medical care
Vitamin C- for skin
Beta carotene- for skin
Ginger

Ear infection:
Beta carotene
Manganese—deficient in ear disorders

Garlic—antimicrobial
Honey--- over a year old only

Edema:
Increase dietary protein, decrease carbohydrate
Chinese parsley
B complex

Emphysema:
Chlorophyll
Omega 3 fatty acids (fish oil)

Endometriosis:
Alfalfa
Astragulus--- antimicrobial
Myrrh
Pau d'arco
Red clover

Fibrocystic breast disorder:
Kelp
Garlic
Shitake
Mullein

Energy:
Wheatgrass
Protein powder
Chlorophyll
Barley grass
Spirulina:
B-12 lozenges—1-5 a day only am

Fever:
Night sweats--- Eliminate dairy from diet or boil dairy at least 20 mins.
Viral or bacterial--- see virus, infection

Flu:
Ginger
Omega 3s --- fish oil
Maitake, Reishi, Shiitake (beta 1,3 glucan)
Wheatgrass
Vitamin C
Aloe Vera

Food poisoning:
Charcoal
Garlic
Potassium

Fracture:
Vitamin C--- makes skin, hair, nail, bone--- 60% protein in body found in bone
Protein
Kelp
Horsetail
Ginger

Fungal infection:
Oregano
Coconut oil—source of capryllic acid
Capryllic acid
Barberry
Oregon grape

Gallbladder disorders:
Digestive enzymes
Alfalfa

GI cleanse:
See Crohns

Hair, nails, skin:
Protein
Lemon, limes, vitamin C
Fish oil
Alfalfa

Headache: (migraine)
Magnesium
Fish oil

Heart:
Tachycardia: magnesium (most common nutritional deficiency)
Check potassium levels---- leafy vegetables
Atherosclerosis:
Lower carbohydrate
Omega 3s-- nature's strongest vasodilator and anti-inflammatory
Vitamin C --- 10 g (2 teaspoons daily)--- best natural chelation therapy
powdered
ginger or comprehensive digestive enzyme
Natokinase

Heartburn:
Chewable papaya
Ginger capsules
Licorice (mucilage)

Heavy metal poisoning:
see mercury

Herpes:
Beta 1,3 d-glucan
l-lysine

HIV:
See viral
See parasite

Infection:
Garlic
Oregano
Olive leaf

Infertility: (male)
Increase protein intake
Selenium
Copper
Lower zinc
Use of Echinacea, Ginkgo and St. Johns Wort can cause infertility
Avoid ulcer medications--- zantac, tagamet

Kidney cleanse:
Hydrangea
Marshmallow root
Black cherry concentrate
B complex
Parsley
Goldenrod
Ginger
Uva ursi
mg citrate
Cranberry
Olive leaf
Black cherry concentrate unsweetened

Liver cleanse:
Complete parasite and kidney cleanse first. See
Detoxification in Resource Section of book for

information on purchasing supplements and cleanse directions.

Ingredients: (Place in container with lid)

Epsom salts: 3and half tablespoons
Olive oil: half cup (virgin olive oil)
Fresh pink grapefruit: 1/2 cup juice. (one may use lemon as well)
Black Walnut Tincture, any strength or 2 freeze-dried capsules: 18 drops (antiparasitic herb)

Take Ornithine: 6 capsules to prevent severe nausea

Menopause:
Omega 3
Lavender oil --- applied to skin (strongly estrogenic—causes gynecomastia in men)

Mercury poisoning:
high dose Vitamin C
comprehensive heavy metal formula
Chinese parsley:

Multiple sclerosis:
Reduced grains
Wheatgrass
Chlorophyll
Detoxification—liver, kidney

Muscle strain, tendonitis, or injury: (or prevention for athletes)
Increase protein intake
Higher Vitamin C intake (squeeze 6 lemons daily, more pepper in diet, supplemental vitamin C if desired)---
primates seek out 6 grams a day of vitamin C as like humans, they produce none on their own, one of the only mammals other than man)

Nasal congestion/cold in infants:
Bed rest, Nasal saline spray, EPA fish oil, fluids, humidifier, healthy foods

Nickel toxicity:
Apple pectin
Garlic
Kelp
High dose Vitamin C chelation IV or long term high dose powder form of vitamin use

Osteoporosis:
Avoid halogens which leech calcium from bones
Fluorine (toothpaste, tap water)
Bromine (bread bleach)
Chlorine (drinking water)
Increase protein (two thirds of collagen in body is found inside bones)
Increase vitamin C

Pain:
Omega 3s--- Twice anti-inflammatory as aspirin
No stomach toxicity

Parasites:
(for unknown cause of fatigue, cancers, and viral diseases)
Parasites in drinking water (giardia can cause lymphomas), dairy, and raw or undercooked fish/meat can contain many varieties of viruses.
(HIV is one type of parasite, a retrovirus carrying liver fluke)

Cloves
Black walnut oil
Wormwood

(most antiparasitic formulas on market contain these three herbs, best taken for 2 months to kill all stages of parasite infestation—worms and larvae)

(See Detoxification in Resources section of book for more information)
Liquid sulfur—for pinworms in children

Parkinson's:
investigate for Lyme disease, see parasite, viral, bacterial, heavy metal
Neuroprotective formula
Omega three (pureDHA)

Pneumonia:
Su and Se
Garlic
Oregano

Polycystic ovarian syndrome:
Lower carbohydrate intake, insulin levels

Pregnancy:
Protein--- deficiency linked to birth defects
Iron 30 mg daily
B complex
Folic acid--- 800 mcg 3 months before pregnancy 1-5 a day. (4mg ok)
Zinc: 15-25 mg daily
Greens formula
Ginger—nausea
Mg-B6 nausea
Mg-Ca – premature contractions or cramps

Premenstrual syndrome:
Omega 3s
Magnesium-B6
EPO
Prostate:
Saw palmetto
Pumpkin seed
Omega 3s
Prostatitis:

Cranberry
Zn6
High PSA—burdock, red clover
Sulfur and selenium

Radiation sickness:
Avoid x-rays
Avoid air travel (one trans-Atlantic flight equals 1 chest x-ray)

Sinusitis:
Garlic
Probiotics
Omega 3s
Bromelain
Ginger
Beta carotene or wheatgrass
Elderberry
Astragulus

Skin:
Vitamin C
Omega 3
Beta carotene or wheatgrass (Retin-A is a vitamin A analogue)
See parasite
See liver

Sunburn:
Low dose vitamin A
Vitamin C
Omega 3 fish oil
Topical aloe Vera

Sleep:
Magnesium or high magnesium vegetable supplement(from wheatgrass, mixed green drink)
Sunflower seed--- lecithin
lower carbohydrate intake before sleep
L-tryptophan--- amino acid
L-theanine
Omega threes
limit medications, limit alcohol, limit calcium (opposite of magnesium)
exercise

Smoking cessation:
B complex
Lecithin

Snake bite:
Magnesium
Charcoal tablets

Stomach:
Mastic gum --- for h. pylori
Probiotics
Licorice root (deglycerinized)
Fiber
Slippery Elm bark
omega 3 fatty acids (fish oil or flax oil)
l-glutamine
bromelain
ginger or papain
vitamin K
avoid unboiled dairy

Thyroid:
Under active: iodine (seaweed, fish), coconut oil, spiraling, avoid radish, cabbage, all soy
Hashimotos---- avoid soy formula and soy products--- leading cause of Hashimotos in Japan (destruction of thyroid) (Babies should never receive soy formula)

Virus:
Ginger or Digestive Enzyme formula
Omega 3s --- fish oil
Maitake, Reishi, Shiitake (beta 1,3 glucans)
Wheatgrass
Vitamin C
Aloe Vera
Spirulina—for lymphocytes
One a day to six a day
Constipating good for diarrhea
Even bacterial
Iodine
Zinc
Elderberry

Vision: (antioxidant)
Beta carotene (greens formula)
Bilberry
Cranberry
Grapeseed
Hawthorn berry

Yeast infection:
Caprylic acid
Coconut oil (source of caprylic acid)
Oregano oil
Low carbohydrate
Vitamin C (for immune system)
Sulfur

Medications and Side Effects

Nervous System

Adrenergic antagonists (alpha, beta blockers):
Arrhythmia, impotence, liver toxicity

Antidepressants:
Tricyclics: cardiotoxicity, convulsions, coma
MAO inhibitors: liver toxicity, convulsions
Serotonin reuptake inhibitors: sexual dysfunction (impotence, impaired ejaculation)

Amphetamines:
psychosis, arrhythmia ,high blood pressure, stroke, cardiac arrest

Cholinergic Agonists:
Parkinson's, AV block, Incontinence

Antipsychotics:
Agranulocytosis of blood cells, motor restlessness, abnormal muscle tone, malignant syndrome, nonreversible involuntary movement of face and extremities, Parkinsonism.

Opioid Analgesics:
respiratory depression, convulsions, impaired learning and memory, addiction and abuse potential

Antianxiety/Insomnia:
slurred speech, clouding of consciousness, coma, respiratory arrest

Anticonvulsants:
decreased IQ and cognition for all

Phenytoin   cleft lip, gingival hyperplasia, hepatotoxic, thrombocytopenia
valproic acid,   neural tube defects in newborns, fatal hepatoxicity in children, agranulocytosis
Ethosuximide hepatotoxicity, lupus, blood dyscrasias

Cardiovascular

Antihypertensives:

Diuretics --- most dangerous class of drugs in addition to Ca blockers
Loop diuretics--- irreversible loss of hearing, Ca toxicity, severe myalgia, kidney damage, electrolyte imbalance
Thiazide diuretics --- impotence, hyperglycemia, GI distress, anuria, hyperuricemia, hypokalemia, severe electrolyte imbalance
Potassium sparing diuretics- hirsutism (hair growth in women), gynecomastia (breast development in men), confusion, fever, vomiting, hyperkaelemia
Osmotic (alcohol)diuretics: headache, confusion, chest pain

Antihypertensives (central anti-adrenergics):

Clonidine—decreased ejaculation, severe depression, hallucinations, sudden dangerous rebound high blood pressure, impotence
Methyldopa—impotence, psychosis, movement disorders, depression
Reserpine, severe depression, irregular heartbeat, Parkinsonism, impotence
Guanabenz—severe rebound high blood pressure, sedation, depression.
Guanethidine—failure to ejaculate, anemia, bradycardia (slow heart beat), muscle tremors, potent orthostatic hypotension (on standing)

Alpha blockers(arteriodilators): (Prazosin) nightmares, sexual dysfunction, electrolyte imbalance, infertility, white blood cell decrease

Beta blockers (heart rate regulators) :

arrhythmia, CNS sedation and depression, impotence, , asthma and bronchospasm, (higher death rate and higher heart attack risk -- Nat Heart, Lung and Blood Institute Cardiac Arrhythmia Suppression Trial)

Vasodilators:

ACE inhibitors: (captopril and similar) reduced white blood cells (neutropenia) and subsequent infections and immune system compromise, intractable cough, anaphylaxis, fetal death in pregnancy, breast enlargement (block aldosterone, a male hormone), liver failure (death), kidney failure, sexual dysfunction.

Angiotensin II antagonists: (losartan and similar)) hypotension, dizziness

Direct vasodilators: *(Minoxidl, Hydralazine, Nitroglycerine) lupus, angina, myocardial infarction, hirsutism, neuritis (nerve pain and inflammation)*

Calcium Channel Blockers: (Filodipine, Diltiazem, Verapamil)
most dangerous class of medications along with diuretics

sexual dysfunction, slow heart beat and eventual Av block, heart attack, dangerously low blood pressure, serious arrhythmias, Gi bleeding, liver and kidney damage

Heart Failure Drugs:
Digoxin, Digitoxin: arrhythmias, visual disturbance, gynecomastia, AV and SA heart block, severe electrolyte imbalance and toxicity with other medications. Low safety index
Bypiridines: GI intolerance, hepatotoxicity, fever, thrombocytopenia

Antiarrythmics:
Class 1a: cinchonism, recurrent arrhythmia, thrombocytopenic purpura, potent anticholinergic effects
Class 1b: weakness, restlessness, seizures, cardiac depression, hepatotoxic
Class 1c: may worsen arrhythmias, may worsen heart failure
Class II (beta blockers)
Class III: life threatening ventricular arrhythmia
Class IV: (calcium channel blockers) sinus bradycardia, AV block, GI upset, left ventricular failure in elderly

Anti-Lipidemics:
Cholestyramine: anemia, ulcers, liver cancer, liver dysfunction
HMG CO A reductase inhibitors: rhabdomyolysis(severe muscle breakdown), severe liver damage (hepatitis and jaundice), nonproduction of steroid hormones (impotence, cancer, insomnia) (Baycol, recalled in 2000 caused over 30 fatalities to rhabdomyolysis—muscle destruction)
Gemfibrozil: liver dysfunction, liver cancer, lupus, impotence

Anticoagulants:
Heparin—hemorrhage, thrombocytopenia
Warfarin—teratogenic, bleeding, necrosis, GI upset

Antithrombotic:
Aspirin-- ulcer, bleeding, hemorrhage

Respiratory

Asthma:
Sympathomimetic bronchodilators (B2 agonists) :
nasal congestion, vasodilation, tachycardia, CNS overstimulation
(mood swings, nightmares), GI abnormalities, tooth discoloration
Methylxanthines-- tachycardia, seizures, brain damage, in high
enough doses fatal
Corticosteroids--- severe glaucoma, osteoporosis, ulcers, Candida
infections, weight gain, insulin resistance, loss of taste or smell,
immune impairment, acne.

Antihistamines:
Ethanolamines i.e. BENADRYL (diphenhydramines, clemastine)
sedation, drowsiness, dizziness, dermatitis, rash, headache, sedation,
decreased libido, impotence, gynecomastia, occasionally blood
dyscrasias, lupus, liver toxicity, renal toxicity, arrhythmia

in some cases fatal heart dysrythmia (Seldane, Hismanal- removed
from market) from severe anticholinergic (bradycardia, arrhythmia,
heart block)

Alkylamines i.e. DIMETANE (Chlorpheniramine,
brompheniramine)
Phenothiazine Promethazine

Loratadine CLARITIN fatal arrhythmias with erythromycin(
pneumonia), ketocanozole (antifungals)

Cold/cough:

Expectorants(Guaifenesin, i.e. Robitussin)—
nausea, vomiting, dizziness
Decongestants:
Pseudoephedrine, i.e. Sudafed, etc.--- high blood pressure, irregular
heartbeat, headache, palpitation.

Phenylpropanolamine (Propagest)---- severely increased risk of stroke

Flu (Influenza virus):

Zanamavir:
colitis, anemia, nosebleed, conjunctivitis.

Cough suppressant: Codeine: codeine is a narcotic and highly addictive, CNS depression, restlessness, hallucinations, convulsions.

Gastrointestinal
Antidiarrheal:
Opiates (Diphenoxylate, Loperamide):
blurred vision, reduced peristalsis, drowsiness, CNS depression,
paralytic ileus
Anticholinergics (Atropine) :
decreased memory, concentration, dry mouth, urinary retention,
tachycardia, Parkinsonism, AV heart block, Incontinence,
Salivation, Lacrimation, Ulceration

Laxatives:
Castor oil: nerve damage, electrolyte imbalance
Bisacodyl, Danthron, Senna, Cascara segrada, Castor Oil
sluggish intestine, dependence, electrolyte loss, dehydration
Lactulose: hepatic encephalopathy, nausea, vomiting
Mineral oil: anal leakage, aspiration pneumonitis
Glycerin: colitis

Ulcer medications:
Metoclopramide (REGLAN) : severe dystonia, restlessness
Histamine blockers:
Cimetidine TAGAMET Ranitidine ZANTAC Famotidine
PEPCID
severe CNS disturbance (dizziness, severe headache), sexual
dysfunction (decreased libido, impotence, gynecomastia), liver toxicity,
kidney toxicity, decreased blood cells, increases toxicity of other drugs
by blocking detoxification in liver.

Proton pump inhibitors:
PRILOSEC Omeprazile, PREVACID Lansoprazole,
NEXIUM (Esomeprazole):
atrophic gastritis, increased susceptibility to infection due to decreased
PH of stomach,
diarrhea, nausea, rash, cough.

Prostaglandins:
Misoprostol – abortion

Antacids:

aluminum salts--- Alzheimers, nervous degeneration, aluminum poisoning

calcium carbonate-- calcium toxicity (nervous headaches, muscle cramps), artherosclerosis, lead poisoning (if from bovine source)

Antibiotics

Penicillins: *Nerrve toxicity (seizures—inhibition of Gaba), depression, irritability ,bloody diarrhea, liver, kidney toxicity, neutropenia and immune depression, anemia, , hypersensitivity (serum sickness, anaphylaxis) , taste abnormality, kidney inflammation*
Amoxicillin:
Nafcillin: severe thrombophlebitis, liver toxicity
Methicillin: coagulopathy
Pipercillin: neutropenia
Vancoymycin: ototoxic (hearing), tachycardia, paresthesias, severe nephrotoxicity
Carbapenems:
(imipenem/Cilastatin) same as penicillin
Monobactams: (aztreonam) similar to penicillin, seizures

Cephalosporins : *anaphylaxis, serum sickness, seizures, neutropenia, thrombocytopenia, anemia, kidney failure, liver abnormalities*

Quinolones, Fluoroquinolones : *hypersensitivity, nausea, seizures, coronary thrombosis, cartilage damage in children, liver toxicity, mild to fatal colitis.*

Aminoglycosides *(gentamycin) : convulsions, irreversible hearing loss, kidney damage, nutrient malabsorption, colitis*

Macrolides *(erythromycin): Hearing loss, colitis, headache*

Lincosamides: *(clindamycin) pseudomembranous colitis*

Tetracyclines: *lupus, esophageal ulcer, very severe nephrotoxicity, very severe hepatotoxicity, increased intracranial pressure, photosensitivity, hernia, colitis*

Antifungals

Amphotericin B low therapeutic index (toxic at every dose), nephrotoxicity, anemia, thrombophlebitis

Ketoconazoles:
hepatic necrosis, gynecomastia (inhibits testosterone synthesis), headache

Griseofulvin: impaired cognition, leucopenia, teratogenic

Terbinafine: neutropenia, skin reactions, eye toxicity

Tuberculosis

Isoniazid hepatitis, hepatotoxicity, neuropathy (B6 deficiency)
Rifampin hepatitis
Pyrizanamide hepatitis, gout
Ethambutol loss of central vision, opthalmalgic disturbances

Antiparasitics

Metronidazole (protozoa) giardia (drinking water), entamoeba histolytica: seizures, ataxia
Lindane seizures, other central nervous disturbance, arrhythmias
Mebendazole (roundworm, pinworm)
Ivermectin

Diabetes

Metformin congestive heart failure, kidney and liver damage, folic acid and vitamin B12 deficiency, nerve damage.

TZDs liver toxicity.

Sulfonylureas Increase insulin levels, increased pancreatic burnout

Insulin replacement therapy Increased risk of Cancer, aggravation of hyperinsulinemia, insulin resistance, and pancreatic burnout in type II diabetes

Osteoporosis:

Fosamax: doubles risk of atrial fibrillation (irregular heartbeat) (Univ. of Washington, Susan Heckbert)

Anaesthesia

Cognitive clouding, impairment, lowered IQ
bladder function loss
paralysis
lupus
loss of sensation
1 in 10,000 mortality in 1980s
Currently closer to 1 in 100,000

local: partial paralysis or loss of muscle, nerve function, loss of sensation

Thiopental sedation, hypnosis, CNS depression, decreased cerebral blood flow, apnea, bronchoconstriction, hypotension, tachycardia, respiratory depression, bronchospasm, anaphylaxis

Propofol bradycardia, hypotension, decreased heart perfusion, apnea, severe cardiovascular depression in elderly

Etomidate: sedation, hypnosis, CNS depression, decreased cerebral blood flow, apnea, bronchoconstriction, hypotension, tachycardia, respiratory depression, bronchospasm, anaphylaxis, mycollonus, vomiting, adrenal insufficiency with chronic use

Ketamine: dissociation or disconnection from surroundings, anesthesia, analgesia, increased intracranial pressure, hallucinations, nightmares

Halothane, enflurane, isoflurane-- malignant hyperthermia, hepatotoxixity, liver failure (halothane) nephrotoxicity (enflurane), storage in fat tissues, respiratory depression,

Medical Procedures

Chemotherapy:

Dr. Hardin Jones-- Medical study shows: untreated patients live up to 4 times longer than those who receive conventional therapy. Patients who refuse chemotherapy and radiation live up to 4 times longer. -- UCa Dept of Medical Physics, Transactions., NY Academy of Science, series 2, v. 18n.3, p. 322

Despite chemotherapy, breast cancer mortality has not changed in the last 70 years. -Thomas Dao, MD NEJM Mar 1975 292 p 707

Medical oncologists recommend chemotherapy for virtually any tumor, with a hopefulness undiscouraged by almost invariable failure. - Albert Braverman M.D. 1991 Lancet 1991 337 p 901

Chemotherapy is basically ineffective in the vast majority of cases in which it is given. Robert Moss, PHD, former Director of Information for Sloan Kettering Cancer Center

Chemotherapy and radiation can increase the risk of developing a second cancer by up to 100 times. -Samuel S. Epstein, Congressional Record, Sept. 9, 1987

Famed biostatistician Ulrich Abel, PHD, also found in a similar 1989 study that "the personal views of many oncologists seem to be in striking contrast to communications intended for the public. -"Chemotherapy report" seasilver.threadnet.com/preventorium/chemo.htm

Because of the problem of nausea and vomiting caused by cancer itself as well as many chemotherapy agents, many cancer patients develop anorexia. It lead to a wasting syndrome called cachexia. It is estimated 40% of patients die of malnutrition rather than the disease itself. www.doctormurray.com/articles/chemotherapy.html

Most cancer patients in this country die of chemotherapy. Chemotherapy does not eliminate breast, colon, or lung cancers. This fact has been documented for over a decade, yet doctors still use chemotherapy. –Dr. Allen Levin, M.D. UCSF The Healing of Cancer

Stanford doctors compared chemotherapy to doing nothing in lymphoma. The patients whose treatment was deferred did just as

well. 23% experience remission lasting 4 months to 6 years.
-"Cheating Fate", Health, April 6, 1992

In the 1994 Journal of the National Cancer Institute, they
published a 47 year study of more than 10,000 patients with
Hodgkin's lymphoma treated with chemotherapy. These patients
encountered an incidence of leukemia six times the normal rate.

Chemotherapy devastates the immune system. Lorraine Day tells
us: Cancer is a disease of the immune system. It's caused by a
depressed immune system. How can it possibly be cured by a
therapy that further damages the immune system? " "Cancer
Doesn't Scare Me Any More—Tim O'Shea in To the Cancer
Patient"

Dr. Ulrich Abel did a comprehensive review of every major review
and analysis of every major study and clinical trial of chemotherapy
ever done. He states that 80% of chemotherapy is worthless and
found the worldwide success rate "appalling". Lancet 10 Aug 91. -
----Tim O'Shea in To the Cancer patient Also "Death by Medicine
at mercola. Com/2003/nov/death_by_medicine.htm"

Radiology:
same as for radiation:
hair loss, cancer, leukemia, lymphoma, impotence, sterility

X- rays: cancer, leukemia, infertility
*CT scan: equivalent of 150 chest x-rays. Highly increased risk of
cancer.*

*Chemotherapy: studies show no improvement in mortality rates with
chemotherapy for breast cancer*

Endocrinology:

Hormone Replacement:
Estrogen: breast cancer
Progesterone: Uterine cancer

Surgical Procedures:

Stomach:
Stomach stapling or partial GI dissection: death from vitamin, mineral, and macronutrient malabsorption and death from infection from tube feeding

Tube or catheter insertions: methicillin resistant staph aureus infection, death

Hysterectomy:
650,000 of 750,000 hysterectomies performed ever year are estimated to be unnecessary ***

Caesareans:
300,000 a year, most unnecessary***

Gallstones:
Another popular surgery that is usually unnecessary

Prostate removal: *declining but still taking place*

Natural Health Resources

Books
Enter The Zone, A Diet by Barry Sears PHD
Diabetes Solution by Richard Bernstein MD
Body Mind Soul by Yitzhak Ginsburg
Transforming Darkness into Light by Y. Ginsburg
Holy Woman by Sarah Rigler
In the Merit of the Righteous Woman by Biale Rebbe
The Reward of the Righetous Woman by Biale Rebbe
Healthy in Mind Body and Spirit (Letters on Health by the
Lubavitcher Rebbe)by Rabbi Sholom B Wineberg

Baby Food
Earth's Best
Hain Celestial Group
4600 Sleepytime Dr.
Boulder, CO 80301
800-434-4246

Homemade Baby
10335 W. Jefferson Blvd
Culver City, CA 90232
800-854-8507

Infant Formula:
Formula is not recommended due to large IQ differences
(40%) in formula-fed and breast-fed infants. Soy formula
is linked to Hashimoto's in infants (retardation) due to its
ant thyroid activity. Over 90% of Hashimoto's in Japan
was traced to soy formula.

Bath Salts:
Dead Sea Bath Salts
PO Box 4118
Chatsworth, CA 91313
Telephone: 818- 717-8300

Breathing:
www.breathdance.org

Cleaning Supplies:
Heather's Oxygen Bleach
Jason Naturals
3515 Eastham Drive
Culver City, CA 90232
310-838- 7543

Sustainable Community Development LLC
PO Box 15155
Kansas City, MO 64106
913-541-9299

Cosmetics:
Bareminerals
Dr. Hauschka
Eminence Organics
Planet Organics
Jurlique
Suki

Craniosacral therapy:
The Upledger Institute, Inc. 800-233-5880
www.upledger.com
Sacoro Occipital Research Society 888-245-1011
www.sorsi.com

Detergents:
Seventh Generation
212 Battery street, Suite A
Burlington, VT 05401

Detoxification Formulas:
Kidney, Liver, Colon, Parasite Detoxification Kits
Purity Products
888-DHC-PURE

Parasite cleanse:
Blessed Herbs 800-489-4372
Ejuva 909-337-5627 www.ejuva.com
Health Force Nutritionals 760-747-8822
www.healthforce.com
Purity 1-888-dhc-pure

Parasite Bioenergy Devices:
www.island.net/-zapper
www.royalrife.com

Dentistry:
Environmental Dental Assoc. 800-388-8124 (for mercury filling removal)
Holistic Dental Assoc. 970-259-1091
www.holisticdental.org
American Academy of Biological Dentistry 408-659-5385
www.biologicaldentistry.org

Digestive Enzymes:
Univase 800-630-4534
Super Power Enzyme 800-446-7462 www.vites.com
Enzymedica 888-918-1118

Energy Healing:
Healing Lev. Healing for Women. www.healinglev.com
Quantum Prayer 888-225-7501
www.energeticbalancing.us
Quantum Distance Healing 866-784-7111
www.distancehealing.net
Rosen Method Movement www.rosenmethod.org
Tools for Wellness 800-449-9887
www.toolsforwellness.com
Intuition Health and Healing www.drjudithorloff.com

Hair Color:
Aubrey Organics
4419 North Manhattan Avenue
Tampa, Fl 33614

Light Mountain
PO Box 1008
Silver Lake, WI 53170
1800 548 3824

Herbs:

Nature's Answer
1-800-439-2324

Eclectic Herbs
36350 SE Industrial Way, Sandy OR 97055
1-800-332-4372

Gaia Herbs
1-800-831-7780

Herbspro.com

Herbalremedies.com
1-866- 467-6744

Heavy Metal Cleanse:
Beyond chelation 800-580-7587 www.longevityplus.net
Oral Chelation formula 800-730-4145 www.natureside
.com
Oral Chelation Plus Formula 800-300-6712
www.extended health.com
American Board of Clinical Metal Toxicology 800-356-
2228 www.abct.info

Herbal Medicine :
Herb Research Foundation 303-449-2265 www.herbs.org
American Botanical Council 512 926 4900
www.herbalgram.org
American Herbal Pharmacopia 831 461 6318
www.herbal-ahp.org

Juicers for Vegetable Juicing
 www.discountjuicers.com

Raw Food World 866-729-3438

Natural Toothpaste, Mouthwash (fluoride-free) :
Tom's of Maine
302 Lafayette Center
Kennebunk, ME 04043
800-FOR-TOMS

Jason Natural Products
4600 Sleepytime Dr.
Boulder, CO 80301   1-877-JASON-01

Full Spectrum Lighting:
Seventh Generation
212 Battery Street Suite A
Burlington, VT 05401

Kosher:
Kosher Organic Meat and Poultry:

Kosher Organic
212-205-1992

SimchaValley Organic Meat
1-866-887-7633

Wise Poultry
Diamond Organics
1272 Highway 1, Moss Landing, California 95039
1888-organic
Available at some Whole Foods

Fresh Fish

AlwaysFreshfish.com

1889 Highway 9 Unit 41
Toms River, NJ 08755
732-349-0518

Vital Choices 800-608 4825

Rosa   877-747-3107
Wild Planet 800- 998-9946

Organic Hormone Free Egg Whites:

Organic Valley (available at Publix)
CROPP Cooperative
One Organic Way
LaFarge, WI 54639
1-888-444-6455

Kosher Vitamins
Sweetwheat Inc (Wheatgrass)
PO Box 187
Clearwater, FL 33757
727-442-5454

Vibrant Health:
Green Vibrance Formula
Green Vibrance for Children
Flax Oil:

Spectrum Organic Oils.
www.spectrumorganics.com
5341 Old Redwood Hwy Ste. 400
Petaluma, CA 94954

Fish Oil:

MarinEpa Vegicap

Liver Cleanse:
Purity Products 1-888-DHC-PURE

802-658-3773 Liver:
Dr. Richard Schulze 800-437-2362 www.dr-schulze.com
Sandra Cabot MD www.liverdoctor .com

Lymph cleanse:
Lymphatic Drainage Practitioners 800-311-9204

Infrared mats   310-799-97111
www.thebestnaturalcures.com
Saunas--- see sauna dealers

Natural Hair and Skin Products:
Burt's Bees, Inc.
633 Davis Drive # 600
Morrisville, NC 27560
www.burtsbees. com

Giovanni Organic Cosmetics
PO Box 6990
Beverly Hills, CA 90212

Naturopathic Physicians:
www.naturopathic. org 866-538-2267
American Holistic Health Assoc. 714-779-6152
www.ahha.org
Bioenergetic Synchronization 888-333-7080

Citizens for Health 612-879-7585 www.citizens. Org

Organic Clothing:

Wild and Wooly Wear 303-642-3144

Mama's Earth 1- 800-620-7388

Harmony Catalog
360 Interlocken Boulevard
Broomfield, CO 80021

Nontoxic Paint:
Harmony Catalog
360 Interlocken Boulevard
Broomfield, CO 80021

Organic Groceries and Products (Canada):
Lady Bug Organic
(Surrey)
604-513-8971

Organic Florida Grapefruit:
(generally December-February)
Harvey's Groves
P.O. Box 560700
Rockledge, Florida 32956
1-800-327-9312

Uncle Matt's Organic
P.O. Box 120187
Clermont, FL 34712
352-394-8737

Hickory Tree Grove
4510 Audubon Avenue
DeLeon Springs, FL 32130.
(386) 985-1655

Pet Food:
Natural Balance High Protein Pet Food
Dick Van Patten's
Natural Balance Pet Foods, Inc.
12924 Pierce Street, Pacoma, CA 91331
1-800-829-4493

Kidney cleanse—after liver cleanse
Purity 1-888-DHC-PURE
Blessed Herbs 800-489-4372
Dr. Richard Schulze 800-437-2362

PH:

Ph Miracle Living 760-751-8321
Ph paper www.discount-vitamins-herbs.com
800-401-9186
PH test strips   877-726-1110
www.thebeewellcompany.com
Universal Supplements 805-646-5936   universal supplements. Com

Reflexology:
Reflexology Association of America 740-657-1695
ww.reflexology-usa.org

Reiki:
Intl. Center for Reiki 800-332-8112 www.reiki.org

Sunscreen:
Aubrey Organics
4419 North Manhattan Avenue
Tampa, Fl 33614

Vitamins

Whole Food Supplements: Only Whole Food Supplements
Are Recommended
Synthetic Vitamins have been shown to increase Cancer
Risk such as Folic Acid
They are no different than pharmaceuticals
Stick to herbal and whole food supplements only,
preferably organic and fresh vegetable juices (wheatgrass,
barleygrass, parsley) available at health food stores

Amazon Herb 866-519-7565
Entiva 800-964-4303
Megafood 800-819-6742
Pure Synergy 800-723-0277
Vitamineral Green 760-747-8822
Gaia Herbs 1-888-917-8269
Nutiva 1-800-993-4367
Health Force Nutritionals 1-800-357-2717

Kosher Whole Food and Herbal based Vitamin Companies
(use expensive, clean, allergy-free whole food ingredients
and greater than 60% are absorbed in whole food form)

Kosher Vitamins: (Certified)
Avoid overpriced synthetic kosher brands and stick to high
quality whole food or herbal companies. Only 10% of
synthetic supplements are absorbed.
Vibrant Health (kosher) Top quality, organic whole food
herbal formulas
Natures Answer (kosher) Large variety of whole food
herbal formulas
Purity 1-888-DHC-Pure (kosher)— Top quality freshest
herbal formulas
Earthrise
NewNutric

Vegicap: (Vegetarian)
Gaia Herbs (vegicap)- Glass bottling

Garden of Life – Top Probiotics and whole food
vegetarian, Glass bottling
Minami MarinEpa Fish Oil—distilled to separate out
omega 6, top quality distilled fish oil
Cold water process distillation
Allergy Research Group (vegicap)—
several high quality formulations are vegicap
cutting edge anti-Cancer formulations
has Physician Advisors - Naturopathic Physicians on staff
highest quality, most expensive sourced ingredients

Vitamin Companies to Avoid:

Any company that uses:
Calcium carbonate- from cows, filled with lead
Glucosamine sulfate from crab (bottom feeders high in toxins)
Soy formula or soy protein powder known to cause hashimotos (mental retardation) in children
Unprocessed fish oils that aren't certified as five star rated fish oils and that don't separate omega 3 (EPA and DHA) from other omega threes and omega sixes.
Whey formulas not from grass fed, hormone free cows
Calcium formulas—leading cause of a heart attack is when calcium breaks off artery
(in brain is known as stroke, in artery known as cardiac arrest) – usually from high sugar
Companies without a licensed nutritionist or Naturopathic Physician on staff
Plastic bottling
Gingko, St. Johns Wort known to cause infertility
Soy lecithin
Bee pollen, known to be a cause of bee population loss in the US
Multilevel marketing companies selling you on a job or career requiring money
Not GMP certified- Good Manufacturing Practices

Environmental Resources:

Social Investing:

www.socialinvest.org/areas/research

Environmentally Friendly Companies:

www.coopamerica.org/programs/responsible

www.responsibleshopper.org

www.glennisgreen.com

Environmental Groups:

Sierra Club www.sierraclub.org

Natural Resources Defense Council

www.nrdc.org/global warming

Paper Saving:

www.newdream.org/junkmail

dmaconsumers.org/offmailinglist.html

Terror Free Gasoline Companies:

BP—British Petroleum

Toxin Exposure Sources:

http://householdproducts.nlm.nih.gov/index.htm.

Top 10 Polluting Companies, 2008

Du Pont
Archer Daniels Midland
Nissan Motors
Bayer
Dow Chemical
Eastman Kodak
General Electric
Arcelor Mittal
US Steel
ExxonMobil

http://www.peri.umass.edu/corporate-toxics.298.0html

Animal Rights Organizations

American Vegan Society
Box H
Malaga, NJ 08328

The Animals Agenda
456 Monroe Turnpike
Monroe, CT 06468

The Animals Voice
PO Box 341347
Los Angeles, CA 90034

The Animal Legal Defense Fund
1363 Lincoln Avenue
San Rafael, CA 94901

Animal Rights Coalitions
Box 214 Planetarium Station
New York, NY 10024

Association of Veterinarians for Animal Rights
15 Dutch St. Suite 500A
New York, NY 10038-3779

Beauty Without Cruelty
175 W 12th St 16G
New York, NY 10011

Between the Species
PO Box 254
Berkeley, CA 94701

CEASE
PO Box 27
Cambridge, MA 02238

Farm Animal Reform Movement
PO box 70123
Washington, DC 20088

The Fund for Animals
200 W 57th street
New York, NY 10019
Humane Farming Association
1550 California Street
San Francisco, CA 94109

The International Primate Protection League
PO Box 766
Summerville, SC 29484

International Society for Animal Rights
421 South State St.
Clarks Summit, PA 18411

National Anti-vivisection Society
53 West Jackson Blvd, Suite 1550
Chicago, IL 60604

Physicians Committee for Responsible Medicine
PO Box 6322
Washington, DC 20015

Psychologists for the Ethical Treatment of Animals
PO Box 87
New Gloucester, ME 04260

Trans-Species Unlimited
PO Box 1553
Williamsport, PA 17703

Trans-Species Unlimited
New York Office
PO Box 20697
Columbus Circle Station
New York, NY 10023

United Action for Animals
205 East 42ndt St.
New York, NY 10013

A Little About the Animals

Birds and Bees

Both birds and bees are especially important to agriculture as pollinators. The development of butterflies is closely linked to the evolution of flowering plants. Almost 80% of flowering plants and most food crops rely on the pollination of birds and bees. These include oils, natural sources of fuel, cotton, spices, and natural medicines. Bees provide us with almonds, alfalfa, tomatoes, chocolate, and coffee. One of every three bites of food we eat is thanks to bees.

In the 1950s, Rachel Carson predicted a "Silent Spring," where the birds never woke, due to the damage caused in the natural food chain by pesticides. We continue to see the effects of pesticides on the number of pollinating bees and birds in many states. Beekeepers in 2007 lost 90% of their hives due to a mysterious malady. Most of our foods, clothing and vital medicines fly on the wings of many birds and bees.

In California today, bees are shipped in every year to pollinate the almonds. Bees have to be shipped from out of state and other countries, because during the other 50 weeks of the year, no bee lives in the almond growing areas due to insufficient plant life to support them. Plant growers have placed such stress on bees that colonies are placed in starvation situations, dying out to disease. The bees brought from countries such as Australia have brought in new diseases, another reason for the sharp decline in bee colonies. This super breeding of "almond" bees is just one of many reasons for the sharp demise of bee colonies. Plant growers have to ensure plant life and food sources are available in the outer lying areas before such type of agriculture is sustainable. Food prices have all increased due to such irresponsible agriculture. Food shortages may be a long term consequence of pesticides, agricultural malpractice, and crop overproduction.

Upwards of 200 million birds are killed each year during migrations by radio, TV and cellular phone towers. Birds carry built in compasses, particles of magnetite in their heads, which allow them to orient to the Earth magnetic field. Purples, greens and blues, trigger their navigational cues. Long, red waves cause them to disorient. Today, the lure of red towers and our mobile phone conversations guide them to a cold and tragic end. Ensuring that we provide for their protection may be vital to our very own adequate food supplies in the future.

Because of decades of warming atmosphere, butterflies and caterpillars are peaking two weeks earlier. In the Netherlands, birds arriving in late April often find no food available for their young by this point in time. Similarly, Emperor Penguin populations, have declined 70% over the past fifty years due to food loss in the warming Antarctic.

Bears

The world population of Polar Bears has declined to 20,000 to 25,000 today because of hunting, and loss of natural habitat and food supplies from global warming. Polar bear is major source of meat for Arctic populations. Some explorers have died from eating polar bear liver which can be so high in Vitamin A as to be deadly. They are currently considered for endangered species protection. During 2007, bears did not enter hibernation in Europe, due to high temperatures. The East Antarctic ice shelf, the largest ice mass on the planet appears to be accelerating its flow into the sea. This is the main reason sea levels have been rising worldwide. Polar bears have been drowning due to melting ice caps. The bears now find themselves having to swim much longer distances from one mass of ice to another. A polar bear can swim 40 miles in search of food. Sometimes the ice can now be more than 40 miles from the shore. A further decrease of their populations by 30% by mid-century is expected if current losses of sea ice continue as rapidly as their current pace .

Elephants

Elephants do share some characteristics in common with humans. They live to reach an age similar to humans about 68-70 years. And they move more gracefully than some might believe considering their enormous size. Small Indian elephants have been domesticated and are considered valuable beasts of burden in parts of the Far East. The elephant adult brain averages 4783 g, the largest among living and extinct terrestrial mammals. Trained elephants have been taught how to paint, balance on a rolling ball or on one foot, perform on a seesaw, ride in jeeps, even play baseball. They are intelligent and compassionate animals. When an elephant dies, the others in its family will gather around it in mourning. When passing by a corpse of a family member they stop as if in memory of their departed. Elephants are some of the few animals known for this practice. In the 1970s and 1980s, deepening African poverty led to large-scale elephant slaughter for ivory trade. Ivory poachers turned places like Tsavo into a killing field. By the 1980's more than half of Africa's 1.3 million elephants were killed.

Tigers

As of 2007, Tigers were classified as endangered with only about 2400 are surviving in the wild, down from 6000 just ten years ago. When tigers are born, cubs are usually born blind. Typically, only one cub of each litter survives. The rapid decline is attributed to both hunting and loss of their natural habitat. Tiger densities in the wild increased moderately in the 1980s because of intensive protection efforts.

Gorillas

The world's gorilla population is relatively small and declining due to hunting, the ravages of Ebola virus, and the pet trade. Only about 600 gorillas are left in the wild, about half of which exist in Rwanda and Uganda. Asia's only ape, the orangutan, is so endangered that many experts believe that it will become extinct in the wild over the next 10 years. The number of apes, many kept as pets, per square kilometer in Taiwan's capital Taipei is now higher than the number of apes in their natural home in the rainforest

Bibliography

i Twain, Mark. Life on the Mississippi. Penguin Putnam. New York, NY. 2001, P.6

iiWilson,Duff.http://www.nytimes.com/2009/03/03/business/03 medschool
iiihttp://www.boston.com/lifestyle/health/articles/2011/07/02/th ree_harvard_psychiatrists_are_sanctioned_over_consulting_fees/

iii Sadur, CN et al. Insulin stimulation of adipose tissue lipoprotein lipase. Use of the euglycemic clamp technique. J Clin Invest 1982 May; 69 (5):1119-1125.

iv. Frayn KN, Coppack SW, Fielding BA, Humphreys SM 1995 Coordinated regulation of hormone-sensitive lipase and lipoprotein lipase in human adipose tissue in vivo: implications for the control of fat storage and fat mobilization. Adv Enzyme Regul 35:163–178

vi Frayn, K.N. Humphreys, Coppack, S.W. Fuel selection in white adipose tissue. Proceedings of the Nutrition Society 54, 177-189.

vii Vaughan M, Steinberg D, Liberman F and Stanley S. Activation and inactivation of lipase in homogenates of adipose tissue. Life Sci 4 1965 (10): 1077-83.

Vii Vaughan, M. The Metabolism of adipose tissue in vivo. J. Lipid Res. 2: 293-316. 1961.

ix Katsumi Iizuka, Bruick, Richard K. Liang, Guosheng, Uyeda, Horton, Jay D. Deficiency of carbohydrate response element-binding protein reduces lipogenesis as well as glycolysis. Proc Natl Acad Sci USA . 2004 May 11; 101(19): 7281-7286.
x Smith and Crouse, 1984 S.B. Smith and J.D. Crouse, Relative contributions of acetate, lactate and glucose to lipogenesis in bovine intramuscular and subcutaneous adipose tissue, Journal of Nutrition 114 (1984), pp. 792–800.
xi Iritani N, Sugimoto T, Fukuda H. Gene expressions of leptin, insulin receptors and lipogenic enzymes are coordinately regulated by insulin and dietary fat in rats. J Nutr. 2000 May;130(5):1183-8.

xii Sachs, Rabbi Jonathan." On Coincidence and Providence." http://www.youtube.com/watch?v=Lds6FklZv-I&feature=related
xiii Foster-Powell, K. et al. International tables of glycemic index, Am J Clin Nutr 1995; 62:871S-93S.

xiv Miller, Janette. Importance of Glycemic Index in Diabetes. Am Journ of Clin Nut. 194, 59 (3): 747S-752S.
xv Flegal KM, Carroll MD, Ogden CL, Johnson CL. Prevalence and Trends in Obesity Among US Adults, 1999-2000. JAMA.2002; 288: 1723-1727.
xvi Eaton, SB. Stone-agers in the fast lane: Chronic degenerative diseases in evolutionary perspective. The American Journal of Medicine. 1988 April; (84):739-749.

xviiPopkin, Barry M, Siega-Riz, Anna Maria. Haines, Pamela S., Jahns, Lisa. Preventive Medicine 32, 245-254 (2001)

xviii Bialostosky K, Wright JD, Kennedy-Stephenson J, McDowell M, Johnson CL. Dietary intake of macronutrients, micronutrients, and other dietary constituents: United States 1988-94. Vital Health Stat 11. 2002 Jul;(245):1-158.
xix Garber A et al. Understanding Insulin Resistance and Syndrome X. Patient Care. June 15, 1996. pp. 198-208.
xx   Kuczmarski RJ, Flegal KM, Campbell SM, Johnson CL. Increasing prevalence of overweight among US adults. The National Health and Nutrition Examination Surveys, 1960 to 1991. JAMA. 1994 Jul 20; 272(3); 205-11/

xxi   Bialostosky K, Wright JD, Kennedy-Stephenson J, McDowell M, Johnson CL. Dietary intake of macronutrients, micronutrients, and other dietary constituents: United States 1988-94. Vital Health Stat 11. 2002 Jul;(245):1-158.
xxii
        Sanson DW. Effects of increasing levels of corn or beet pulp on utilization of low-quality crested wheatgrass hay by lambs and in vitro dry matter disappearance of forages. J Anim Sci. 1993 Jun;71(6):1615-22.
xxiii   Herrera E, Amusquivar E. Lipid metabolism in the fetus and the newborn. Diabetes Metab Res Rev. 2000 May-Jun;16(3):202-10

xxiv
        Gabbe SG et al. Fetal carbohydrate metabolism: its clinical importance. Am J Obstet Gynecol 1977 Jan 1; 127 (1) : 92-103
xxv   Michal et al. Glucose Tolerance and excessively large infants. A twelve-year follow-up study. Am J obset Gynecol. 1966 Jan 1: 94.

xxvi   Mayor F, Cuezva JM. Biol Neonate. 1985;48(4):185-96.Hormonal and metabolic changes in the perinatal period.

xxvii   Ozanne, Se, Hales CN. The long-term consequences of intra-uterine protein malnutrition for glucose metabolism. Proc Nutr Soc. 1999 Aug;58(3):615-9.

xxviii   Clinton takes aim at child obesity. http://www.cbsnews.com/stories/2005/05/03/health/main69276 7.shtml
xxix   http://www.nal.usda.gov/fnic/foodcomp/cgi-bin/list_nut_edit.pl
xxx   Richard AF, Dewer RE Lemur Ecology Ann Rev Ecol Sys 22: 145-175. (1991)
xxxi   Hawkes, K. , Hill, K. and O'Connel, JF. (1981). Why hunters gather:optimal foraging and the Ache of Eastern Paraguay. American Ethnologist.
xxxii   Hill, Kim. Hunting and Human Evolution. Journal of Human Evolution (1982) 11, 521-544.
xxxiii   Ramakrishnan et al.
xxxiv   Hill, Kim. Hunting and human evolution. Journal of Human Evolution. 11, 521-544. 1982.
xxxv   Walker, Alexander. Nutrition, diet, physical activity, smoking, and longevity. From primitive hunter-gatherer to present passive consumer- how far can we go. Nutrition 19 (2) Feb 2003, 1699-173.
xxxvi   Leonard, William R. FOOD for thought. Scientific American 287 no6 106-15 D 2002

xxxvii   Hill, Kim. Hunting and Human Evolution. Journal of Human Evolution (1982) 11, 521-544.

xxxviii   Hill, Kim. Hunting and human evolution. Journal of Human Evolution. 11, 521-544. 1982.
xxxix——Cordain L, Miller JB, Eaton SB, Mann N, Holt SH, Speth JD. Plant-animal subsistence ratios and macronutrient energy estimations in worldwide hunter-gatherer diets. Am J Clin Nutr. 2000 Mar;71(3):682-92.
xl   Milton, Katharine. Diet and Primate Evolution. Scientific American, August 1993. PP??????
xli   Hill, Kim. Hunting and human evolution. Journal of Human Evolution. 11, 521-544. 1982.
xlii
xliii   Hill, Kim. Hunting and Human Evolution. Journal of Human Evolution (1982) 11, 521-544.

xliv   Walker, Alexander. Nutrition, diet, physical activity. p.5
xlv   Walker, Alexander. Nutrition, diet, physical activity. p. 5.
xlvi
http://www.csun.edu/science/health/docs/tv&health.html
xlvii Rilke, Rainer Maria. Letters to a Young Poet. WW Norton. New York. 1993.
xlviii   Wilson, Christina The ultimate question book Smithsonian 2006 Harper Collins Publishers.

xlix   Levey, Douglass J., Martinez Del Rio, Carlos. It takes guts (and more) to eat fruit: Lessons from Avian Nutritional Ecology. The Auk 118 (4): 819-831, 2001.

l   Podlesak DW, McWilliams SR. Metabolic routing of dietary nutrients in birds: effects of diet quality and macronutrient composition revealed using stable isotopes. Physiol Biochem Zool. 2006 May-Jun;79(3):534-49. Epub 2006 Apr 6.

li   McWilliams, Scott R., Karasov, William H. Phenotypic flexibility in digestive system structure and function in migratory birds and its ecological significance. Comparative biochemistry and Physiology Part A 128 (2001) 579-593.
lii   Suthers, Hannah B, Bickal, Jean M, Rodewald, Paul G. Use of Successional Habittat and Fruit Resources by Songbirds during Autumn Migration in Central New Jersey. Wilson Bull, 112 (2), 2000, pp. 249-260.
liii   Gannes, Leonard Z. comparative fuel use of migrating passerines: Effects of fat stores, migration distance, and diet. The Auk 118(3):665-677, 2001.
liv   Weidensaul, Scott. Living on the Wind Across the Hemisphere with Migratory Birds. P.112. North Point Press. New York, NY. 1999.
lv   McGranahan, Devan Allen, Kuiper, Shonda, Brown, Jonathan M. temporal Patterns in use of an Iowa Woodlot During the Autumn Bird migration. Am. Midl. Nat. 153:61-70.
lvi   Weidensaul, Scott. Living on the Wind. P. 6 North Point Press. New York, NY. 1999.
lvii   Cunningham et al. Encyclopedia.....
lviii   Battley PF. Adaptations for endurance exercise in migratory birds. Asia Pac J Clin Nutr. 2003;12 Suppl:S3.
lix   Bairlein, Franz. Migration: Energetics. Encyclopedia of Life Sciences 2002, John Wiley and sons, Ltd. www.els.net.

lx http://www.enchantedlearning.com/subjects/butterflies/allabout/
lxi   Levey, Douglass J., Martinez Del Rio, Carlos. It takes guts (and more) to eat fruit: Lessons from Avian Nutritional Ecology. The Auk 118 (4): 819-831, 2001.
lxii   Babile, R.; Auvergne, A.; Delpech, P.; et al. Evolution de la consommation de mais au cours du gavage et incidence sur la production de foie gras chez le canard de Barbarie.Annales de Zootechnie (Paris) 36 (1) : 73-83 : 1987
lxiii   Levey, Douglass J et al. It takes guts…
lxiv   Hargrove, James L. Adipose energy stores, physical work, and the metabolic syndrome: lessons from hummingbirds. Nutrition Jounral 2005, 4:36. pp.1-5.
lxv   Greenewalt, Crawford H., Hummingbirds. Dover Publications. New York, 1990. pp. 9-11.
lxvi   McGranahan, Devan Allen, Kuiper, Shonda, Brown, Jonathan M. temporal Patterns in use of an Iowa Woodlot During the Autumn Bird moigration. Am. Midl. Nat. 153:61-70.
lxvii   Persson IL, Wikan S, Swenson JE, et al. The diet of the brown bear Ursus arctos in the Pasvik Valley, northeastern Norway. Wildlife Biology. 7 (1): 27-37 Mar 2001.
lxviii   Rue III
lxix   Benson, John f. Chamberlain, Michael J. food Habits of Louisiana Black Bears in two subpopulations of the Tensas river basin. The American Midland Naturalist. 156 (1) July 2006. 118-127.
lxx   2 Auger, Janene, Meyer, Susan E., Black L. Hal. Are American Black Bears (Ursus americanus) Legitimate Seed Dispersers for Fleshy-fruited Shrubs?The American Midland Naturalist. Volume 147, Issue 2 (April 2002) pp. 352–367

lxxi   Grenfell W. E., A. J. Brody. 1983. Seasonal foods of black bears in Tahoe National Forest, California. California Fish and Game. 69:132–150.

lxxii   Raine R. M., J. L. Kansas. 1990. Black bear seasonal food habits and distribution by elevation in Banff National Park, Alberta. International Conference on Bear Research and Management. 8:297–304.

lxxiii   Richardson W. S. 1991. Habitat selection and feeding ecology of black bears in southeastern Utah. M.Sc. Thesis, Brigham Young University, Provo, Utah. 75 p.

lxxiv   Persson IL, Wikan S, Swenson JE, et al. The diet of the brown bear Ursus arctos in the Pasvik Valley, northeastern Norway. Wildlife Biology. 7 (1): 27-37 Mar 2001.
lxxv   Richardson 1991.

lxxvi   Rue III
lxxvii   Rue III
lxxviii   Haroldson, Mark A., Schwartz, Charles C., Cherry, Steve, Moody, David S. Possible effects of elk harvest on fall distrivution of grizzly bears in the greater Yellowstone ecosystem. Journal of Wildlife Management 68 1) Jan 2004. pp. 129-137.
lxxix   Rue III
lxxx   Persson IL, Wikan S, Swenson JE, et al. The diet of the brown bear Ursus arctos in the Pasvik Valley, northeastern Norway. Wildlife Biology. 7 (1): 27-37 Mar 2001.
lxxxi   Persson IL, Wikan S, Swenson JE, et al. The diet of the brown bear Ursus arctos in the Pasvik Valley, northeastern Norway. Wildlife Biology. 7 (1): 27-37 Mar 2001.
lxxxii   Wood, Daniel. Bears. Whitecap Books. Vancouver, Canada. 1995.

lxxxiii   Aichun, X, Zhigang, Jiang, Chunwang, Li, Jixun, Guo, Guosheng, Wu, Ping, Cai. Summer Food habits of brown bears in Kekexili Nature Reserve, Ainghai-Tibetan plateau, China. 17 (2) Nov 2006. 132-137.
lxxxiv   Goldstein, Isaac, Paisley, Susanna, Wallace, Robert, Jorgenson, Jeffrey P., Cuesta, Francisco, Castellanos, Armando. Andean bear-livestock conflicts: a review. 17 (1) April 2006.
lxxxv   Swenson, J.E., Jansson, A., Riig, R. and Sandegren, F., 1999. Bears and ants: myrmechophagy by brown bears in central Scandinavia. Can. J. Zool. 77, pp. 551–561
lxxxvi   Rue III
lxxxvii   Smith, Tom S., Partridge, dynamics of Intertidal foraging by Coastal Brown Bears in Soutwestern Alaska. Journal of Wildlife Management. 68 (2) April 2004. pp. 233-240.
lxxxviii   Robbins, Charles T, Schwartz, Chrles C., Felicetti, Laura A. , Nutritional ecology of ursids: a review of newer methods and management implications. 15 (2: Nov 2004. 161-171.
lxxxix   Hilderbrand, GV, Jenkins SG, Hanley TA, and Robbins CT. Effect of seasonal differences in dietary meat intake on changes in body mass and composition in wild and captive brown bears. Canadian Journal of Zoology 77: 1999.:1623-1630.
xc   Cutin, Charles B.

xci   Rue III
xcii   Cutin, Charles B.
xciii   Rue III
xciv   Rue III
xcv   Smil, Vaclav. Vaclav Smil (2002) Eating Meat: Evolution, Patterns, and Consequences Population and Development Review 28 (4), 599–639.
xcvi   Cuvelier, C. , Clinquart, A., Hocquette, JF, Cabaraux, JF. Dufrasne, I. Istasse, L. Hornick, JL. Comparison of composition and quality traits of meat from young finishing bulls from Belgian Blue, Limousin and Aberdeen Angus breeds. Meat Science 74 (2006) 522-531.
xcvii   Campling, R.C. Processing cereal grains for cattle—a review. Livestock Production Science, 28 (1991) 223-234.
xcviii Broadbent PJ. A note on the effect of omitting the cereal supplement from a finishing diet offered to weaned single suckle calves. Animal Production. 24(2). 1977. 275-278.
xcix   Hidiroglou, N., McDowell, LR, Johnson, DD. Effect of Diet on Animal Performance, Lipid composition of Subcutaneous Adipose and Liver Tissue of Beef Cattle. Meat Science 20 (19877) 195-210.
c   Robinson, DL, Oddy, VH. Genetic parameters for feed efficiency, fatness, muscle area and feeding behaviour of feedlot finished beef cattle. Livestock Production Science 90 (2004) 255-270.
ci   Hadjipanayiotou, Replacement of soybean meal and barley grain by chicpeas in lamb and kid fattening diets. Animal Feed Science Technology 96 (2002) 103-109.
cii   Bacvanski, S. Maize grain or ears in concentrate diets for young fattening bulls. Animal Feed Science Technology, 1 (1976) 393-400.
ciii   Bodas, R. Giraldez, FJ, Lopez, S., Rodriguez, AB, Mantecon, AR. Inclusion of sugar beet pulp in cereal-based diets for fattening lambs. Small Ruminant Research (2006), doi:10.1016/j.smallrumres.2006.07.006.
civ   M. S. Zaman, Z. Mir, P. S. Mir, A. El-Meadawy, T. A. McAllister, K. -J. Cheng, D. ZoBell and G. W. Mathison Performance and carcass characteristics of beef cattle fed diets containing silage from intercropped barley and annual ryegrass Animal Feed Science and Technology, Volume 99, Issues 1-4, 30 August 2002, Pages 1-11

cv   Sanson DW. Effects of increasing levels of corn or beet pulp on utilization of low-quality crested wheatgrass hay by lambs

and in vitro dry matter disappearance of forages. J Anim Sci. 1993 Jun;71(6):1615-22.
cvi   Christine Janis, "Artiodactyla", in AccessScience@McGraw-Hill, http://www.accessscience.com, DOI 10.1036/1097-8542.053500, last modified: July 15, 2002.
cvii   Langer, P. Evidence from the digestive tract on phylogenetic relationships in ungulates and whales. J Zool Syst Evol Research 39 (2001) 77-90.
cviii   Christine Janis, "Artiodactyla", in AccessScience@McGraw-Hill, http://www.accessscience.com, DOI 10.1036/1097-8542.053500, last modified: July 15, 2002.

cix   Bodas, R. Giraldez, FJ, Lopez, S., Rodriguez, AB, Mantecon, AR. Inclusion of sugar beet pulp in cereal-based diets for fattening lambs. Small Ruminant Research (2006), doi:10.1016/j.smallrumres.2006.07.006.
cx   Spears, Jerry W. Beef Nutrition in the 21st century. Animal Feed Science Technology 58 (1996) 29-35.
cxi   Bodas, R. Giraldez, FJ, Lopez, S., Rodriguez, AB, Mantecon, AR. Inclusion of sugar beet pulp in cereal-based diets for fattening lambs. Small Ruminant Research (2006), doi:10.1016/j.smallrumres.2006.07.006.
cxii   Singer, Peter. Animal Liberation. 2002. Harper Collins. New York. P. 140.
cxiii   Mann NJ. Asia Pac J Clin Nutr. 2004;13(Suppl):S17.Paleolithic nutrition: what can we learn from the past?

cxiv   Carrington, Richard. Elephants A Short Account of their Natural History Evolution and Influence on Mankind. 1959 Basic Books Inc. New York. p.67

cxv

http://www.shemayisrael.co.il/publicat/hazon/tzedaka/elephant.h

tm

cxvi   Codron, Jacqui, Lee-Thorp, Julia A., Sponheimer, Matt, Codron, David, Grant, Rina C., De Rutter, Darryl J. Elephant Diets in Kruger National Park, South Africa: Spatial and Landscape Differences. Journal of Mammalogy, 87(1):27-34, 2006.
cxvii   Codron, Jacqui, Lee-Thorp, Julia A., Sponheimer, Matt, Codron, David, Grant, Rina C., De Rutter, Darryl J. Elephant

Diets in Kruger National Park, South Africa: Spatial and Landscape Differences. Journal of Mammalogy, 87(1):27-34, 2006.
cxviii   Codron, Jacqui, Lee-Thorp, Julia A., Sponheimer, Matt, Codron, David, Grant, Rina C., De Rutter, Darryl J. Elephant Diets in Kruger National Park, South Africa: Spatial and Landscape Differences. Journal of Mammalogy, 87(1):27-34, 2006.
cxix   Codron, Jacqui, Lee-Thorp, Julia A., Sponheimer, Matt, Codron, David, Grant, Rina C., De Rutter, Darryl J. Elephant Diets in Kruger National Park, South Africa: Spatial and Landscape Differences. Journal of Mammalogy, 87(1):27-34, 2006.
cxx   Codron, Jacqui, Lee-Thorp, Julia A., Sponheimer, Matt, Codron, David, Grant, Rina C., De Rutter, Darryl J. Elephant Diets in Kruger National Park, South Africa: Spatial and Landscape Differences. Journal of Mammalogy, 87(1):27-34, 2006.
cxxi   Class m, Frey r, Kiefer b, Lechner-doll m, Loehlein w, Polster c, Tossner ge, Streich wj. The maximum attainable body size of herbivorous mammals: morphophysiological constraints on foregut, and adaptations of hindgut fermenters. Oecologia 2003 (136): 14-27.
cxxii   Codron, Jacqui, Lee-Thorp, Julia A., Sponheimer, Matt, Codron, David, Grant, Rina C., De Rutter, Darryl J. Elephant Diets in Kruger National Park, South Africa: Spatial and Landscape Differences. Journal of Mammalogy, 87(1):27-34, 2006.
cxxiii   Rue III, Leonard Lee. Sportsman Guide to Game Animals. Harper and Row. 1968. p. 567
cxxiv   Sues, Hans-Dieter, Reisz, Robert R. Origins and early evolution of herbivory in tetrapods. Tree 1998: 13 (4) : 141-145.
cxxvYoung V, Pellett P (1994) "Plant proteins in relation to human protein and amino acid nutrition." American Journal of Clinical Nutrition, vol. 59(suppl), pp. 1203S-1212S.

cxxvi   Hill, Kim. Hunting and human evolution. Journal of Human Evolution. 11, 521-544. 1982.
cxxvii   Tallas, Peter G, White, Robert G. Glucose Turnover and defense of Blood glucose levels in arctic foz. Comp. biochem. Physiol vol 91 A, No. 3, pp. 493-498, 1988.
cxxviii   Bradshaw, Evolutionary...
cxxix
         Bradshaw CJ, Hindell MA, Best NJ, Phillips KL, Wilson G, Nichols PD. You are what you eat: describing the foraging ecology of southern elephant seals (Mirounga leonina) using blubber fatty acids.
Proc Biol Sci. 2003 Jun 22;270(1521):1283-92.
cxxx

Bradshaw CJ, Hindell MA, Best NJ, Phillips KL, Wilson G, Nichols PD. You are what you eat: describing the foraging ecology of southern elephant seals (Mirounga leonina) using blubber fatty acids. Proc Biol Sci. 2003 Jun 22;270(1521):1283-92.
cxxxi
Shah P, Isley WL. N Engl J Med. 2006 Jan 5;354(1):97-8. Ketoacidosis during a low-carbohydrate diet..
cxxxii
Shah P, Isley WL. N Engl J Med. 2006 Jan 5;354(1):97-8. Ketoacidosis during a low-carbohydrate diet..

cxxxiii   Tallas et al.
59   cxxxiv   Bevier WC, Jovanovic-Peterson L, Formby B, Peterson CM. Maternal hyperglycemia is not the only cause of macrosomia: lessons learned from the nonobese diabetic mouse Am J Perinatol. 1994 Jan;11(1):51-6.

cxxxv   Bradshaw, John WS, Goodwin, Deborah, Legrand-Defretin, Veronique, Nott, Helen M.R. Food Selection by the Domestic Cat, an Obligate Carnivore. Comp. Biochem. Physiol. 1996. 114A(3): 205-209.
cxxxvi   Macdonald ML, Rogers QR, Morris JG. Nutrition of the domestic cat, a mammalian carnivore. Annu Rev Nutr. 1984;4:521-62.

cxxxvii   Kienzle E. Blood sugar levels and renal sugar excretion after the intake of high carbohydrate diets in cats. J Nutr. 1994 Dec;124(12 Suppl):2563S-2567S.

cxxxviii   Bradshaw, John WS, Goodwin, Deborah, Legrand-Defretin, Veronique, Nott, Helen M.R. Food Selection by the Domestic Cat, an Obligate Carnivore. Comp. Biochem. Physiol. 1996. 114A(3): 205-209.
cxxxix   Bradshaw, JWS, Horsfield, GF, Allen, JA, Robinson, IH, Feral cats: their role in the population dynamics of Felis catus. Applied Animal Behaviour Science. Dec 1999; Vol 65(3):273-283.
cxl   Bradshaw, The Evolutionary Basis for the feeding behavior of Domestic Dogs (Canis familiaris) and Cats (Felis catus) 1-3. the Jounral of Nutrition. Bethesda: Jull 2006. (136), 7s:1927-1932.
cxli   Tallas et al.
cxlii   Tallas, Peter G, White, Robert G. Glucose Turnover and defense of Blood glucose levels in arctic fox. Comp. biochem. Physiol vol 91 A, No. 3, pp. 493-498, 1988.

cxliii   Belo, PS, Romsos, DR, and Leveille, GA, 1976. Influence of diet on glucose tolerance, on the rate of glucose utilization and on gluconeogenic enzyme activities in the dog. J. Nutr. 106, 1465-1474.
cxliv   National Geographic. Vol 13. p.52 2007.
cxlv   Bradshaw, Evolutionary...
cxlvi   Zuberbuhler, Klaus, Jenny, David. Leopard predation and primate evolution. Journal of Human Evolution (2002) 43, 873-886.
cxlvii   Verheagen et al.
cxlviii   Lawick-Goodall 1968
cxlix   Gladikas-Brindamour(1)

cl   Fossey D, Harcourt AH (1977) "Feeding ecology of free-ranging mountain gorilla (gorilla gorilla beringei)." In: Primate Ecology: Studies of Feeding and Ranging Behaviour in Lemurs, Monkeys, and Apes, ed. Clutton-Brock TH; Academic Press, New York, pp. 415-447.

cli   Chivers 1972
clii   Dart, RA Carnivorous propensities of baboons. Symp. zool. Soc. Lond. 10:49-56. (1963)
cliii   Breur, Thomas, Diet choice of large carnivores in northern Cameroon. Afr J Ecol, 43, 181-90.
cliv   Altmann, SA, and Altmann, J Baboon Ecology: African Field Research. Chicago: University of Chicago Press. 1970
clv   Hamilton, WJ III, and Busse, CD Primate carnivory and its significance to human diets. Bio. Sci.28:761-766. 1978
clvi   Harding, RSO, Predation by a group of olive baboons (Papio Anubis). Am J Phys. Anthropol. 38:587-592. 1973
clvii   Hausfater, G Predatory behavior of yellow baboons. Behaviour 56:44-68. 1976.
clviii   Weisman, Alan. The World Without Us. P. 87
clix   Boesch C, Boesch H Hunting behavior of wild chimpanzees in the Tai National Park. am J Phys Anthropol 78:547-573. 1989
clx   Mills, MGL, Biggs HC Prey apportionment and related ecological relationships between large carnivores in Kruger National Park. Mammals as Predators, pp 253-268. Oxford: Clarendon Press.
clxi   Stanford CB, Wallis J, Matama H, Goodall HJ Patterns of predation by chimpanzees on red colobus monkeys in Gombe National Park, 1982091. Am J Phys Anthropol 94: 213-228. 1994.
clxii

clxiii   Hill, Kim. Hunting and Human Evolution. Journal of
Human Evolution. 111982. 521-544..
clxiv Donnelly, John. Boston Globe November 13, 2006
Hemmed in by burgeoning settlement in Tanzania, apes are
dying off; the Jane Goodall Institute has a strategy to save
them.
http://www.boston.com/news/globe/health_science/articles
/2006/11/13/of_chimps_and_humans/ Of chimps and
humans
clxv   Pilbeam DR. Genetic and morphological records of the
Hominoidea and hominid origins: a synthesis. Molecular Phylogeny
and Evolution 5:155-168. 1996.
clxvi   Begun, David R. Relations Among the great Apes and
Humans: New Interpretations Based on the fossil great ape
dryopithecus. Yearbook of Physical Anthropology 37:11-63 (1994)
clxvii   Begun DR. Relations among the great apes and humans.
Yearbook of Physical Anthropology 37: 11-63. 1994.
clxviii   Begun Dr. Miocene fossil hominids and the chimp-
human clade. Science. 1992 Sep 25;257(5078):1929-33.
clxix   Weisman, Alan. The World Without Us. P. 50.
clxx   Marroig, Gabriel, Cheverud, James M. Size as a line of
least evolutionary resistance: diet and adaptive morpholoigical
radiation in new world monkeys. Evolution. 2005 May; 59(5):1128-
1142.
clxxi   Goodman, Morris, Grossman, Lawrence I, Wildman,
Derek E. Moving primate genomics beyond the chimpanzee
genome. trends in genetics. Vol. 21 No. 9 Sep 2005.
clxxii   Marroig, Gabriel, Cheverud, James M. Size as a line of
least evolutionary resistance: diet and adaptive morpholoigical
radiation in new world monkeys. Evolution. 2005 May; 59(5):1128-
1142.
clxxiii   Narita Y, Oda S, Takenaka O, Kageyama T. Multiplicities
and some enzymatic characteristics of ape pepsinogens and pepsins.
J Med Primatol 2000; 29; 402-410.
clxxiv   http://www.indiana.edu/~primate/primates.html

clxxv   Foley RA, Lee PC, Ecology and Energetics of
encephalization in hominid evolution. Philos Trans R Soc Lond B
Biol Sci. 1991 Nov 29;334(1270):223-31
clxxvi   Smil, Vaclav. Eating meat: Evolution, Patterns, and
Consequences.
clxxvii

Garber AJ. New standards to reduce morbidity and mortality in hospitalized patients with diabetes. Am Fam Physician. 2006 Feb 15; 73(4): 591, 594.

clxxviii Despres JP et al. Hyperinsulinemia as an independent risk factor for ischemic heart disease. NEJM 1996; 334:952-957.
clxxix
Ford, ES et al. Risk factors for mortality from all causes and from coronary heart disease among persons with diabetes. findings from the National Health and Nutrition examination Survey I Epidemiologic Follow-up Study. Am J Epidemiol 1991 Jun 15; 133(12): 1220-1230.
clxxx
Laakso M. Epidemiology of diabetic dyslipidemia. Diabetes Rev 1995;3:408-22.
clxxxi Basciano H, Federico L, Adeli K. Fructose, insulin resistance, and metabolic dyslipidemia. Nutr Metab (Lond). 2005 Feb 21;2(1):5.

clxxxii Fagot –Campana, A. Emergence of Type II Diabetes in Children.The Epidemiological Evidence. J Pediatr Endocrinol Metab. (in press)
clxxxiii Demetriou K, H'Maltezou E, Pierides AM. Familial homozygous hypercholesterolemia: effective long-term treatment with cascade double filtration plasmapheresis. Blood Purif. 2001;19(3):308-13.

clxxxiv Yuan G. Wang J Hegele RA. Heterozygous familial hypercholesterolemia: an underrecognized cause of early cardiovascular disease. CMAJ. 2006 Apr 11;174(8):1124-9.5(2): 147.
clxxxv Kume S, Takeya M, Mori T, Araki N, Suzuki H, Horiuchi S, Kodama T, Miyauchi Y and Takahashi K. Immunohistochemical and ultrastructural detection of advanced glycosylation end products in atherosclerotic lesions of human aorta with a novel specific monoclonal antibody. American Journal of Pathology, MONTH" 1995 147, 654-667.

clxxxvi Dagogo-Jack S. Preventing diabetes-related morbidity and mortality in the primary care setting. J Natl Med Assoc. 2002 Jul;94(7):549-60.

clxxxvii Romeo JH, Seftel AD, Madhun ZT, Aron DC. Sexual function in men with diabetes type 2: association with glycemic control. J Urol. 2000 Mar;163(3):788-91.

clxxxviii
    Morrison J et al. Effect of high glucose on gene
expression in mesangial cells: upregulation of the thiol pathway is
an adaptational response. Physiol Genomics. 2004
clxxxix   Chiu CJ, Milton RC, Gensler G, Taylor A. Association
between dietary glycemic index and age-related macular
degeneration in nondiabetic participants in the Age-Related Eye
Disease Study.
Am J Clin Nutr. 2007 Jul;86(1):180-8.
cxc   Monnier V. M., Kohn R. R., Cerami A. Accelerated age-
related browning of human collagen in diabetes mellitus. Proc. Natl.
Acad. Sci. U.S.A. 1984; 81:583-587

cxci   Uesugi N et al, Possible mechanism for medial smooth
muscle cell injury in diabetic nephropathy: glycoxidation-mediated
local complement activation. Am J Kidney Dis. 2004 Aug;
44(2):224-38.

cxcii   McPherson J. D., Shilton B. H., Walton D. J. Role of
fructose glycation and cross-linking of proteins. Biochemistry 1988;
27:1901-1907

cxciii   Levi B, Werman MJ. Long-term fructose consumption
         accelerates glycation and several age-related variables in male
         rats.J Nutr. 1998 Sep;128(9):1442-9.

cxciv   Levi B, Werman MJ. J Nutr. 1998 Sep;128(9):1442-9.
Long-term fructose consumption accelerates glycation and several
age-related variables in male rats.

cxcv   Paul R. G., Bailey A. J. Glycation of collagen: the basis of
its central role in the late complications of ageing and diabetes. Int.
J. Biochem. Cell Biol. 1996; 28:1297-1310.
cxcvi
         74 Soininen K, Niemi M, Kilkki E, Strandberg T, Kivisto
KT. Muscle symptoms associated with statins: a series of twenty
patients. Basic Clin Pharmacol Toxicol. 2006 Jan;98(1):51-4.

cxcvii   Andrejak M, Gras V, Caron J. Severe muscle disorders
associated with statins: analysis of cases notified in France up to the
end of February 2002 and data concerning the risk profile of
cerivastatin. Therapie. 2005 May-Jun;60(3):299-304.

cxcviii   Al-Jubouri MA, Young RM. Hypertriglyceridaemia: a pointer to diabetes mellitus and alcoholism.
Ann Clin Biochem. 1993 Mar;30 (Pt 2):201-2.

cxcix   Thabet MA, Salcedo JR, Chan JC. Hyperlipidemia in childhood nephrotic syndrome.
Pediatr Nephrol. 1993 Oct;7(5):559-66.

cc   Levy E, Thibault L, Turgeon J, Roy CC, Gurbindo C, Lepage G, Godard M, Rivard GE, Seidman E. Beneficial effects of fish-oil supplements on lipids, lipoproteins, and lipoprotein lipase in patients with glycogen storage disease type I.
Am J Clin Nutr. 1993 Jun;57(6):922-9.

cci   Weisman, Alan. The World Without Us. p. 146.
ccii
cciii   Singer, Peter. Animal Liberation. Harper Collins. New York. 2002. P. 168
cciv   Gore, Al. An Inconvenient Truth. Rosedale Publishing, New York, NY. p.58.
ccv   Gore, Al. An Inconvenient Truth. Rosedale Publishing. 2007. p. 164.
ccvi   Pollak et al. 2010
ccvii   Pollak et al 2010
ccviii   Gambineri, Allessandra, Pelusi Carla, Manicardi Elisa, Vicennati Velentina, Cacciari Mauro, Morselli-Labate, Antonio Maria, Pagotto, Uberto, Pasquali, Renato. Glucose intolerance in a large cohort of Mediterranean women with polycystic ovary syndrome. Diabetes 53 2004 Sept : 53 (9): 2353-2358.
ccix   Pelusi B, Gambineri A, Pasquali R. Type 2 diabetes and the polycystic ovary syndrome.
Minerva Ginecol. 2004 Feb;56(1):41-51.
ccx   Nestler JE, Stovall D, Akhter N, Iuorno MH and Jakubowicz, DJ. Strategies for the use of insulin-sensitizing drugs to treat infertility in women with polycystic ovary dyndrome. Fertil Steril 77 (2001), pp. 209-215.
ccxi   Ganmaa, D. Wang, PY, Qin, LQ, Hoshi, K, Sato, A. Is Milk responsible for male reproductive disorders? Medical Hypotheses 2001 57 (4), 510-514.
ccxii   Ganmaa, D. Wang, PY, Qin, LQ, Hoshi, K, Sato, A. Is Milk responsible for male reproductive disorders? Medical Hypotheses 2001 57 (4), 510-514.
ccxiii   Ganmaa, D. Wang, PY, Qin, LQ, Hoshi, K, Sato, A. Is Milk responsible for male reproductive disorders? Medical Hypotheses 2001 57 (4), 510-514.

ccxiv   Weisman, Alan. The World Without Us. P. 125.
ccxv   Weisman, Alan. The World Without Us. P. 74, 116.
ccxvi   Weisman, Alan. The World Without Us. P. 139
ccxvii   (JAMA April 15, 1998;279(15):1200-5)
ccxviii Nurs Times. December 9-15, 2003;99(49):24-5.
ccxix   Pharm World Sci December, 2003;25(6):264-8.
ccxx   J Clin Pharm Ther   October, 2000;25(5):355-61   J Am
Geriatr Soc   December, 2002;50(12):1962-8
ccxxi   http://www.rain-tree.com/facts.htm
ccxxii   Singer, Peter. Animal Liberation. 2002. Harper Collins.
New York. P. 167
ccxxiii http://www.rain-tree.com/facts.htm
ccxxiv   Speth, John D. Early hominid hunting and scavenging: the
role of meat as an energy source. Journal of Human Evolution
(1989) , 18, 329-343.
ccxxv
http://news.independent.co.uk/environment/article2081668.ece.
Lean, Geoffrey, 10 years to live: Orangutan faces extinction in the
wild The Independent/blogs. 17 December 2006

ccxxvi   Carl Safina, Carl, Rosenberg, Andrew A., Myers,
Ransom A, Quinn II, Terrance J, Collie, Jeremy S. U.S. Ocean
Fish Recovery: Staying the Course Science 29 July 2005: Vol. 309.
no. 5735;707 - 708
ccxxvii   Singer, Peter. Animal Liberation, Harper Collins. New
York, NY. 2002. P. 37.
ccxxviii Revkin, Andrew C. NY Times.com/dotearth. New
Times Postings p. D8 Jan. 6, 2009
ccxxix   http://library.thinkquest.org/26823/agriculture.htm
ccxxx   Layman, Donald K, Baum, Jamie I. 2004 Dietary protein
impact on glycemic control during weight loss.   The American
Society for Nutritional Sciences J. Nutr. 134:968S-973S, April 2004.

ccxxxi Rabbi Ben Tzion Krasnianski. Lecture 2011.
ccxxxii Gretah, Smadar. www.smadarshulamit.com. Energy Healing for
Women. 2012
ccxxxiii Rabbi Yaakov Yagen. Lecture. 2011.
ccxxxiv Rabbi Ben Tzion Krasnianski. Lecture 2011.
www.Chabaduppereastside.com
ccxxxv Rebbetzin Esther Jungreis. Lecture, www.Hineni.org 2012.
ccxxxvi Rabbi Yisroel Jungreis. Lecture, www.Hineni.org. 2012.
ccxxxvii Rabbi Yaakov Yagen. www.yaakovcares.com. Lecture 2011.

ccxxxix Rabbi Ben Tzion Krasnianski.Lecture. 2012.

ABOUT THE AUTHOR

Dr. Sarlin pursued medical studies in England and received his M.D. degree from Xavier College of Medicine, completing his clinical rotations in Atlanta, Georgia. He received his Masters of Nutrition from Columbia University College of Physicians and Surgeons. He studied Medical Sciences for one year at Sackler University in Tel Aviv, Israel and received his Bachelors from Cornell University in Literature. He currently practices Naturopathic Medicine and Nutrition and lives in New York City.

Printed in Great Britain
by Amazon.co.uk, Ltd.,
Marston Gate.